HIGH-PR PLANT-BASED Cookbook FOR ATHLETES

Many **High-Protein Vegan** and **Vegetarian Recipes** to Boost your Body **to the TOP!**

The Best **220+** Green and Healthy Recipes to **Perform your Muscles** and **Sculpt your Abs** stay LIGHT!

2 BOOKS IN 1

By
William Miller

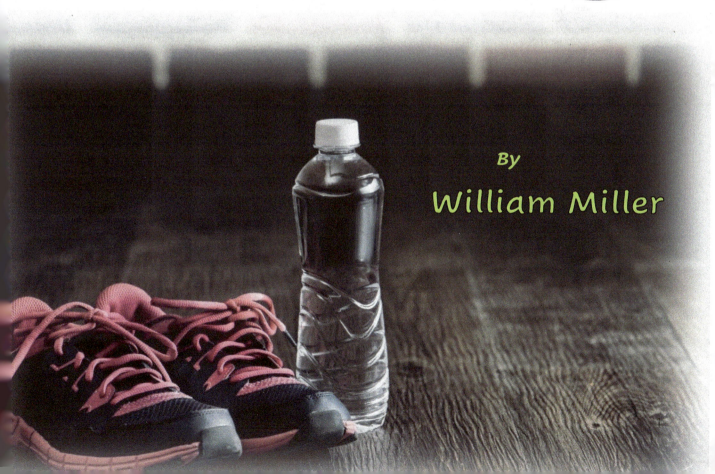

Table of Contents

Introduction 5
BOOK 1: THE PLANT-BASED FOR MEN 7
Chapter 1. BREAKFAST AND SNACKS 8
1) Frittata with Mushrooms and Peppers 9
2) frozen Hemp and Blackberry Smoothie Bowl 9
3) dark Chocolate and Walnut Steel-Cut Oats 9
4) easy Buckwheat Porridge with Apples-Almonds 10
5) traditional Spanish Tortilla 10
6) special Chocolate and Mango Quinoa Bowl 10
7) easy Orange and Carrot Muffins with Cherries 11
8) simple Quinoa Lemony Muffins 11
9) rich Oatmeal Almond Porridge 11
10) rich Breakfast Pecan and Pear Farro 11
11) simple Blackberry Waffles 12
12) authentic Walnut Waffles with Maple Syrup 12
13) simple Orange and Bran Cups with Dates 12
14) exotic Macadamia Nuts and Apple-Date Couscous 12
15) tasty Blueberry Coconut Muffins 13
16) Swiss-style Chard Scrambled Tofu 13
17) best Baked Spicy Eggplant 13
18) very good Mashed Broccoli with Roasted Garlic 13
19) simple Spicy Pistachio Dip 14
20) hungarian Paprika Roasted Nuts 14
21) easy Mixed Vegetables with Basil 14
22) delicious Onion Rings and Kale Dip 14
23) Portuguese Soy Chorizo Stuffed Cabbage Rolls 15
24) tropical Banana Tangerine Toast 15
25) easy Maple Banana Oats 15
26) tasty Gingerbread Belgian Waffles 16
27) easy Banana and Walnuts Porridge 16
Chapter 2. LUNCH 17
28) italian Mushroom Soup of Medley 18
29) mediterranean Dill Cauliflower Soup 18
30) special Fennel Broccoli Soup 18
31) easy Bean Soup Asian-Style 19
32) Tortilla Mexican-style Soup 19
33) hot Bean Spicy Soup 19
34) special Mushroom Rice Wine Soup 19
35) tasty Bean Tangy Tomato Soup 20
36) easy Spinach and Potato Soup 20
37) mexican Bean Turmeric Soup 20
38) tropical Coconut Arugula Soup 21
39) authentic Lentil Soup with Swiss Chard 21
40) autumn Spicy Farro Soup 21
41) all Colored Chickpea Salad 22
42) Mediterranean-style Lentil Salad 22
43) delicious Roasted Avocado and Asparagus Salad 22
44) special Green Bean Cream Salad with Pine Nuts 23
45) easy Kale Cannellini Bean Soup 23
46) delicious Mushroom Soup with Hearty Cream 23
47) Italian-style Authentic Panzanella Salad 24
48) asian Black Bean Quinoa Salad 24
49) moroccan Power Bulgur Salad with Herbs 24
50) authentic Roasted Pepper Salad 25
51) autumn Hearty Quinoa Soup 25
52) special Green Lentil Salad 25
53) easy Chickpea, Acorn Squash, and Couscous Soup 26
54) special Pumpkin Cayenne Soup 26
55) easy Zucchini Cream Soup with Walnuts 26
56) traditional Ramen Soup 27
57) mexican Black-Eyed Pea Soup 27
58) greek Leeks Cauliflower Soup 27
59) italian Lentil Lime Soup 27
60) asian Rice, Spinach, and Bean Soup 28
61) Creamy Potato Soup with Herbs 28
62) 28
63) asian Quinoa and Avocado Salad 28
64) vegetarian Tabbouleh Salad with Tofu 29
65) special Green Pasta Salad 29
Chapter 3. DINNER 30
66) authentic Ukrainian Borscht 31
67) moroccan Lentil Beluga Salad 31
68) Indian-style Naan Salad 31
69) italian Broccoli Ginger Soup 32
70) asian Noodle Rice Soup with Beans 32
71) special Vegetable and Rice Soup 32
72) easy Daikon and Sweet Potato Soup 32
73) tasty Chickpea and Vegetable Soup 33
74) Italian-style Bean Soup 33
75) lovely Brussels Sprouts and Tofu Soup 33
76) creamy White Bean Rosemary Soup 34
77) delicious Mushroom and Tofu Soup 34
78) tropical Coconut Cream Butternut Squash Soup ... 34
79) italian Mushroom Coconut Soup 34
80) greek Tomato Cream Soup 35
81) special Roasted Pepper Salad in Greek-Style 35
82) sweet Potato and Kidney Bean Soup 35
83) winter Quinoa Salad with Pickles 36
84) super Wild Roasted Mushroom Soup 36
85) special Green Bean Soup in Mediterranean-Style 36
86) lovely Creamy Carrot Soup 37
87) special Italian Nonno's Pizza Salad 37
88) special Cream of Golden Veggie Soup 37
89) easy Roasted Cauliflower Soup 38
90) authentic Vegan Coleslaw 38
91) super Hot Collard Salad 38
92) super Roasted Mushrooms and Green Beans Salad 39
93) mexican Bean and Couscous Salad 39
94) vegetarian Seitan and Spinach Salad a la Puttanesca 39
95) pomodoro and Avocado Lettuce Salad 40
96) special Fried Broccoli Salad with Tempeh and Cranberries 40
97) healthy Balsamic Lentil Salad 40
98) super Hot Green Bean and Potato Salad 40
99) easy Millet Salad with Olives and Cherries 41
100) delicious Daikon Salad with Caramelized Onion 41
101) Black cabbage and beet salad 41
102) Pomodoro Lettuce Salad 42
103) Avocado Arugula Salad 42
Chapter 4. DESSERTS 43
104) Southern american Apple Cobbler with Raspberries 44
105) sweet Chocolate Peppermint Mousse 44
106) tasty Raspberries Turmeric Panna Cotta 44
107) spring Banana Pudding 45
108) everyday Baked Apples Filled with Nuts 45
109) summer Mint Ice Cream 45
110) tasty Cardamom Coconut Fat Bombs 45
111) hungarian Cinnamon Faux Rice Pudding 46
112) sweet White Chocolate Fudge 46
113) italian Macedonia Salad with Coconut and Pecans 46
114) authentic Berry Hazelnut Trifle 46
115) vegetarian Avocado Truffles with Chocolate Coating ... 47
116) delicious Vanilla Berry Tarts 47
117) best Homemade Chocolates with Coconut and Raisins 47
118) simple Mocha Fudge 47
119) east Almond and Chocolate Chip Bars 48
120) Almond Butter Cookies 48
BOOK 2: THE PLANT-BASED DIET COOKBOOK 49
Chapter 1. BREAKFAST AND SNACKS 50
121) american Kentucky Cauliflower with Mashed Parsnips 51
122) spanish Spinach Chips with Guacamole Hummus 51
123) super Buttered Carrot Noodles with Kale 51
124) healthy Parsley Pumpkin Noodles 52
125) easy Mixed Vegetables with Basil 52
126) delicious Onion Rings and Kale Dip 52
127) Portuguese Soy Chorizo Stuffed Cabbage Rolls 52
128) asian Sesame Cabbage Sauté 53
129) pomodori Stuffed with Chickpeas and Quinoa 53
130) Herbed Vegetable Traybake 53
131) american Louisiana-Style Sweet Potato Chips 53
132) special Bell Pepper and Seitan Balls 54
133) italian Parmesan Broccoli Tots 54
134) tasty Chocolate Bars with Walnuts 54
135) simple Carrot Energy Balls 55
136) super Crunchy Sweet Potato Bites 55
137) best Roasted Glazed Baby Carrots 55
138) everyday Oven-Baked Kale Chips 56

139)	special Cheesy Cashew Dip	56
140)	healthy Peppery Hummus Dip	56
141)	original Lebanese Mutabal	56
142)	best Indian-Style Roasted Chickpeas	57
143)	easy Avocado with Tahini Sauce	57
144)	healthy Sweet Potato Tater Tots	57

Chapter 2. LUNCH 58

145)	best Braised Kale with Sesame Seeds	59
146)	autumn Roasted Vegetables	59
147)	authentic Moroccan Tagine	59
148)	Chinese-style Cabbage Stir-Fry	60
149)	special Sautéed Cauliflower with Sesame Seeds	60
150)	best Sweet Mashed Carrots	60
151)	lovely Sautéed Turnip Greens	60
152)	asian Yukon Gold Mashed Potatoes	61
153)	super Aromatic Sautéed Swiss Chard	61
154)	typical Sautéed Bell Peppers	61
155)	classic Mashed Root Vegetables	61
156)	easy Roasted Butternut Squash	62
157)	classical Sautéed Cremini Mushrooms	62
158)	easy Roasted Asparagus with Sesame Seeds	62
159)	special Greek-Style Eggplant Skillet	62
160)	simple Cauliflower Rice	63
161)	simple Garlicky Kale	63
162)	vegetarian Tofu Cabbage Stir-Fry	63
163)	special Smoked Tempeh with Broccoli Fritters	63
164)	simple Cheesy Cauliflower Casserole	64
165)	very Spicy Veggie Steaks with Green Salad	64
166)	mexican-style Jalapeño Quinoa Bowl with Lima Beans	64
167)	itaian Black-Eyed Pea Oat Bake	64
168)	hungarian Paprika Fava Bean Patties	65
169)	simple Walnut Lentil Burgers	65
170)	asian Couscous andQuinoa Burgers	65
171)	special Bean and Pecan Sandwiches	65
172)	simple Homemade Kitchari	66
173)	Piccante Green Rice	66
174)	special Asian Quinoa Sauté	66
175)	italian Farro and Black Bean Loaf	66
176)	special Cuban-Style Millet	67
177)	classic Cilantro Pilaf	67
178)	typical Oriental Bulgur andWhite Beans	67
179)	Red Lentils with Mushrooms	67
180)	special Colorful Risotto with Vegetables	68
181)	easy Amaranth Grits with Walnuts	68
182)	delicious Barley Pilaf with Wild Mushrooms	68
183)	tasty Sweet Cornbread Muffins	69
184)	italian Acrylic Rice Pudding with Dried Figs	69
185)	simple Potage au Quinoa	69
186)	easy Sorghum Bowl with Almonds	69

Chapter 3. DINNER 70

187)	simple Cauliflower Rice	71
188)	simple Garlicky Kale	71
189)	italian Artichokes Braised in Lemon and Olive Oil	71
190)	mediterranean Rosemary and Garlic Roasted Carrots	71
191)	easy Mediterranean-Style Green Beans	72
192)	simple Roasted Garden Vegetables	72
193)	quick Roasted Kohlrabi	72
194)	special Cauliflower with Tahini Sauce	72
195)	italian-style Herb Cauliflower Mash	73
196)	best Garlic and Herb Mushroom Skillet	73
197)	simple Pan-Fried Asparagus	73
198)	easy Gingery Carrot Mash	73
199)	only Mediterranean-Style Roasted Artichokes	74
200)	asian Thai-Style Braised Kale	74
201)	special Silky Kohlrabi Puree	74
202)	tasty Creamy Sautéed Spinach	74
203)	best Tofu Skewers with Salsa Verde and Squash Mash	75
204)	special Mushroom Lettuce Wraps	75
205)	original Garlicky Rice	75
206)	classic Brown Rice with Vegetables and Tofu	75
207)	simple Amaranth Porridge	76
208)	classic Country Cornbread with Spinach	76
209)	simple Rice Pudding with Currants	76
210)	easy Millet Porridge with Sultanas	76
211)	english Quinoa Porridge with Dried Figs	77
212)	easy Bread Pudding with Raisins	77
213)	simple Bulgur Wheat Salad	77
214)	quick Rye Porridge with Blueberry Topping	77
215)	exotic Coconut Sorghum Porridge	78
216)	mamma's Aromatic Rice	78
217)	Everyseasons Savory Grits	78
218)	only Greek-Style Barley Salad	78
219)	special Sweet Maize Meal Porridge	79
220)	delicious Dad's Millet Muffins	79
221)	simple Ginger Brown Rice	79
222)	everyday Chili Bean and Brown Rice Tortillas	79
223)	easy Cashew Buttered Quesadillas with Leafy Greens	80
224)	everyday Asparagus with Creamy Puree	80
225)	simple Kale Mushroom Galette	80
226)	genovese Focaccia with Mixed Mushrooms	81
227)	vegetarian Seitan Cakes with Broccoli Mash	81
228)	special Spicy Cheese with Tofu Balls	81
229)	tasty Quinoa andVeggie Burgers	81
230)	easy Baked Tofu with Roasted Peppers	82
231)	simple Zoodle Bolognese	82
232)	special Zucchini Boats with Vegan Cheese	82
233)	special Roasted Butternut Squash with Chimichurri	82

Chapter 4. DESSERTS 83

234)	milk Chocolate Fudge with Nuts	84
235)	not too sweet Chocolate and Peanut Butter Cookies	84
236)	special Mixed Berry Yogurt Ice Pops	84
237)	everyday Holiday Pecan Tart	84
238)	tropical Coconut Chocolate Barks	85
239)	easy Nutty Date Cake	85
240)	delicious Berry Cupcakes with Cashew Cheese Icing	85
241)	exotic Coconut and Chocolate Cake	85
242)	italian Berry Macedonia with Mint	86
243)	special Cinnamon Pumpkin Pie	86
244)	everytime Party Matcha and Hazelnut Cheesecake	86
245)	italian Pistachios and Chocolate Popsicles	87
246)	english Oatmeal Cookies with Hazelnuts	87
247)	tropical Coconut Chocolate Truffles	87
248)	delicious Layered Raspberry and Tofu Cups	87
249)	easy Cashew and Cranberry Truffles	88
250)	Coconut Peach Tart	88
251)	tropical Mango Muffins with Chocolate Chips	88
252)	easy Maple Rice Pudding	88
253)	delicious Vanilla Cookies with Poppy Seeds	89
254)	best Kiwi and Peanut Bars	89
255)	special Tropical Cheesecake	89
256)	english Raisin Oatmeal Biscuits	89
257)	exotic Coconut and Chocolate Brownies	90
258)	rich Everyday Energy Bars	90
259)	healthy Raw Coconut Ice Cream	90
260)	delicious Chocolate Hazelnut Fudge	90
261)	english Oatmeal Squares with Cranberries	90

Bibliography 91
Conclusion 92

© **Copyright 2021 - All rights reserved.**

The content contained within this book may not be reproduced, duplicated or transmitted without direct written permission from the author or the publisher.

Under no circumstances will any blame or legal responsibility be held against the publisher, or author, for any damages, reparation, or monetary loss due to the information contained within this book. Either directly or indirectly.

Legal Notice:

This book is copyright protected. This book is only for personal use. You cannot amend, distribute, sell, use, quote or paraphrase any part, or the content within this book, without the consent of the author or publisher.

Disclaimer Notice:

Please note the information contained within this document is for educational and entertainment purposes only. All effort has been executed to present accurate, up to date, and reliable, complete information. No warranties of any kind are declared or implied. Readers acknowledge that the author is not engaging in the rendering of legal, financial, medical or professional advice. The content within this book has been derived from various sources. Please consult a licensed professional before attempting any techniques outlined in this book.

By reading this document, the reader agrees that under no circumstances is the author responsible for any losses, direct or indirect, which are incurred as a result of the use of information contained within this document, including, but not limited to, — errors, omissions, or inaccuracies.

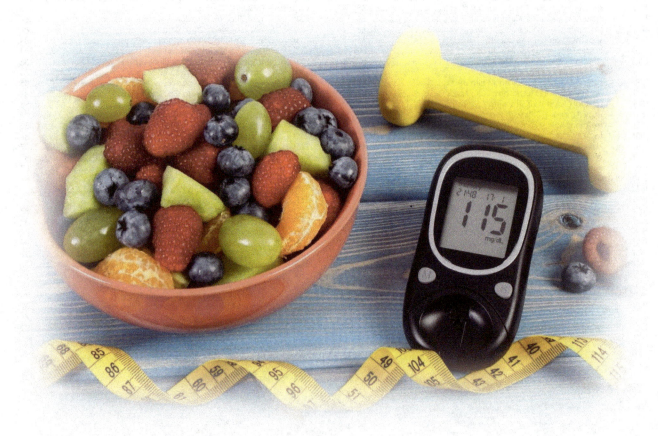

Introduction

Have you ever wondered what is good for our bodies?

Have you ever wondered what foods we humans should really be eating?

Most importantly: do you ever make a list of the foods you eat just to count the junk and tell yourself "it will get better next week?"

In recent years, people have become increasingly concerned about what they eat.
It is important to eat healthy foods, without preservatives or additives, to provide the right nutrients to the body.
Scientists say to eat natural and minimally processed foods, and in this only one diet meets this need: **the Plant-Based Diet!**
The Plant-Based Diet is based on *fruits*, *vegetables* and *nuts*, without any nutritional intake from animal protein.

But why should a person follow the Plant-Based Diet?

Clinical studies show that in ancient times, humans ate mainly harvested foods that grew wild on the ground. This is also evidenced by our teeth: they are more similar to herbivorous animals, which use them to grind nuts or chew herbs for long periods of time, than those of carnivores, which use them to tear and tear meat from the body of their prey.
Thanks to this growing body of information and proven clinical studies, people are increasingly interested in eating less processed foods, and this trend has turned many people into vegetarians or even vegans.

The Plant-Based diet allows you to get the right amount of nutrients and follow an eating plan that makes you light and fit, that's why it's the best solution!

The Plant-Based diet is suitable for everyone: kids, over 50, women, men and even for beginners! In my opinion **everybody should follow the plant-based diet**, and this is why I have created a book series on the Plant-Based diet specific for each category of people!

Specifically, due to this diet allows the body to work well, staying fit and Light, the Plant-based diet is perfect for **ATHLETES!**

"High-Protein Plant-Based for Athletes Cookbook", indeed, is a collection of the best recipes of 2 of my favorite books: "The Plant-Based diet for Men Cookbook" and "The Plant-Based diet Cookbook" to give all my readers more than 220 fantastic and simple recipes for accompanying their fitness!

Are you ready to discover the best 220 Plant-Based recipes for Athletes? GO!

BOOK 1: THE PLANT-BASED FOR MEN

Chapter 1. BREAKFAST AND SNACKS

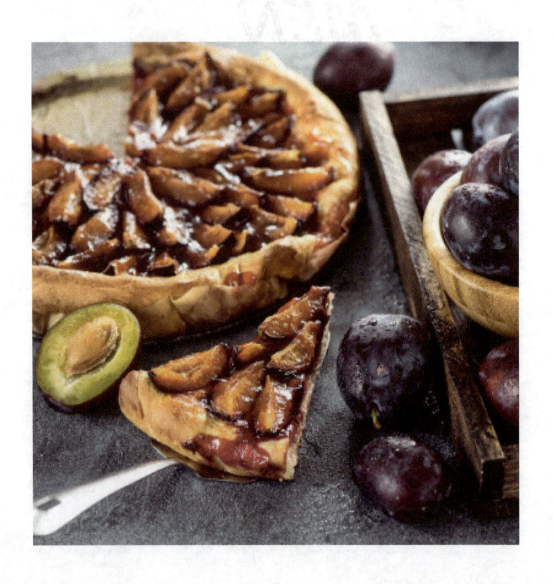

1) FRITTATA WITH MUSHROOMS AND PEPPERS

Preparation Time: 30 minutes | **Servings:** 4

Ingredients:
- 4 tbsp olive oil
- 1 red onion, minced
- 1 red bell pepper, sliced
- 1 tsp garlic, finely chopped
- 1 pound button mushrooms, sliced
- Sea salt and ground black pepper, to taste
- 1/2 tsp dried oregano
- 1/2 tsp dried dill
- 16 ounces tofu, drained and crumbled
- 2 tbsp nutritional yeast
- 1/2 tsp turmeric powder
- 4 tbsp corn flour
- 1/3 cup oat milk, unsweetened

Directions:
- Preheat 2 tbsp of the olive oil in a nonstick skillet over medium-high heat. Then, cook the onion and pepper for about 4 minutes until tender and fragrant.
- Add in the garlic and mushrooms and continue to sauté an additional 2 to 3 minutes or until aromatic. Season with salt, black pepper, oregano and dill. Reserve.
- In your blender or food processor, mix the tofu, nutritional yeast, turmeric powder, corn flour and milk. Process until you have a smooth and uniform paste.
- In the same skillet, heat 1 tbsp of the olive oil until sizzling. Pour in 1/2 of the tofu mixture and spread it with a spatula.
- Cook for about 6 minutes or until set; flip and cook it for another 3 minutes. Slide the omelet onto a serving plate.
- Spoon 1/2 of the mushroom filling over half of the omelet. Fold the unfilled half of omelet over the filling.
- Repeat with another omelet. Cut them into halves and serve warm. Enjoy

2) FROZEN HEMP AND BLACKBERRY SMOOTHIE BOWL

Preparation Time: 10 minutes | **Servings:** 2

Ingredients:
- 2 tbsp hemp seeds
- 1/2 cup coconut milk
- 1 cup coconut yogurt
- 1 cup blackberries, frozen
- 2 small-sized bananas, frozen
- 4 tbsp granola

Directions:
- In your blender, mix all ingredients, trying to keep the liquids at the bottom of the blender to help it break up the fruits.
- Divide your smoothie between serving bowls.
- Garnish each bowl with granola and some extra frozen berries, if desired. Serve immediately

3) DARK CHOCOLATE AND WALNUT STEEL-CUT OATS

Preparation Time: 30 minutes | **Servings:** 3

Ingredients:
- 2 cups oat milk
- 1/3 cup steel-cut oats
- 1 tbsp coconut oil
- 1/4 cup coconut sugar
- A pinch of grated nutmeg
- A pinch of flaky sea salt
- 1/4 tsp cinnamon powder
- 1/4 tsp vanilla extract
- 4 tbsp cocoa powder
- 1/3 cup English walnut halves
- 4 tbsp chocolate chips

Directions:
- Bring the oat milk and oats to a boil over a moderately high heat. Then, turn the heat to low and add in the coconut oil, sugar and spices; let it simmer for about 25 minutes, stirring periodically.
- Add in the cocoa powder and continue simmering an additional 3 minutes.
- Spoon the oatmeal into serving bowls. Top each bowl with the walnut halves and chocolate chips.
- Enjoy

4) EASY BUCKWHEAT PORRIDGE WITH APPLES-ALMONDS

Preparation Time: 20 minutes

Servings: 3

Ingredients:
- 1 cup buckwheat groats, toasted
- 3/4 cup water
- 1 cup rice milk
- 1/4 tsp sea salt
- 3 tbsp agave syrup
- 1 cup apples, cored and diced
- 3 tbsp almonds, slivered
- 2 tbsp coconut flakes
- 2 tbsp hemp seeds

Directions:
- In a saucepan, bring the buckwheat groats, water, milk and salt to a boil. Immediately turn the heat to a simmer; let it simmer for about 13 minutes until it has softened.
- Stir in the agave syrup. Divide the porridge between three serving bowls.
- Garnish each serving with the apples, almonds, coconut and hemp seeds. Enjoy

5) TRADITIONAL SPANISH TORTILLA

Preparation Time: 35 minutes

Servings: 2

Ingredients:
- 3 tbsp olive oil
- 2 medium potatoes, peeled and diced
- 1/2 white onion, chopped
- 8 tbsp gram flour
- 8 tbsp water
- Sea salt and ground black pepper, to season
- 1/2 tsp Spanish paprika

Directions:
- Heat 2 tbsp of the olive oil in a frying pan over a moderate flame. Now, cook the potatoes and onion; cook for about 20 minutes or until tender; reserve.
- In a mixing bowl, thoroughly combine the flour, water, salt, black pepper and paprika. Add in the potato/onion mixture.
- Heat the remaining 1 tbsp of the olive oil in the same frying pan. Pour 1/2 of the batter into the frying pan. Cook your tortilla for about 11 minutes, turning it once or twice to promote even cooking.
- Repeat with the remaining batter and serve warm

6) SPECIAL CHOCOLATE AND MANGO QUINOA BOWL

Preparation Time: 35 minutes

Servings: 2

Ingredients:
- 1 cup quinoa
- 1 tsp ground cinnamon
- 1 cup non-dairy milk
- 1 large mango, chopped
- 3 tbsp unsweetened cocoa powder
- 2 tbsp almond butter
- 1 tbsp hemp seeds
- 1 tbsp walnuts
- ¼ cup raspberries

Directions:
- In a pot, combine the quinoa, cinnamon, milk, and 1 cup of water over medium heat. Bring to a boil, low heat, and simmer covered for 25-30 minutes. In a bowl, mash the mango and mix cocoa powder, almond butter, and hemp seeds. In a serving bowl, place cooked quinoa and mango mixture.
- Top with walnuts and raspberries. Serve immediately

7) EASY ORANGE AND CARROT MUFFINS WITH CHERRIES

Preparation Time: 45 minutes **Servings:** 6

Ingredients:
- 1 tsp vegetable oil
- 2 tbsp almond butter
- ¼ cup non-dairy milk
- 1 orange, peeled
- 1 carrot, coarsely chopped
- 2 tbsp chopped dried cherries
- 3 tbsp molasses
- 2 tbsp ground flaxseed
- 1 tsp apple cider vinegar
- 1 tsp pure vanilla extract
- ½ tsp ground cinnamon
- ½ tsp ground ginger
- ¼ tsp ground nutmeg
- ¼ tsp allspice
- ¾ cup whole-wheat flour
- 1 tsp baking powder
- ½ tsp baking soda
- ½ cup rolled oats
- 2 tbsp raisins
- 2 tbsp sunflower seeds

Directions:
- Preheat oven to 350 F. Grease 6 muffin cups with vegetable oil.
- In a food processor, add the almond butter, milk, orange, carrot, cherries, molasses, flaxseed, vinegar, vanilla, cinnamon, ginger, nutmeg, and allspice and blend until smooth.
- In a bowl, combine the flour, baking powder, and baking soda. Fold in the wet mixture and gently stir to combine. Mix in the oats, raisins, and sunflower seeds. Divide the batter between muffin cups. Put in a baking tray and bake for 30 minutes

8) SIMPLE QUINOA LEMONY MUFFINS

Preparation Time: 25 minutes **Servings:** 5

Ingredients:
- 2 tbsp coconut oil melted, plus more for coating the muffin tin
- ¼ cup ground flaxseed
- 2 cups unsweetened lemon curd
- ½ cup pure date sugar
- 1 tsp apple cider vinegar
- 2 ½ cups whole-wheat flour
- 1 ½ cups cooked quinoa
- 2 tsp baking soda
- A pinch of salt
- ½ cup raisins

Directions:
- Preheat oven to 400 F.
- In a bowl, combine the flaxseed and ½ cup water. Stir in the lemon curd, sugar, coconut oil, and vinegar. Add in flour, quinoa, baking soda, and salt. Put in the raisins, be careful not too fluffy.
- Divide the batter between greased with coconut oil cups of the tin and bake for 20 minutes until golden and set. Allow cooling slightly before removing it from the tin. Serve

9) RICH OATMEAL ALMOND PORRIDGE

Preparation Time: 25 minutes **Servings:** 4

Ingredients:
- 2 ½ cups vegetable broth
- 2 ½ cups almond milk
- ½ cup steel-cut oats
- 1 tbsp pearl barley
- ½ cup slivered almonds
- ¼ cup nutritional yeast
- 2 cups old-fashioned rolled oats

Directions:
- Pour the broth and almond milk in a pot over medium heat and bring to a boil. Stir in oats, pearl barley, almond slivers, and nutritional yeast. Reduce the heat and simmer for 20 minutes. Add in the rolled oats, cook for an additional 5 minutes, until creamy. Allow cooling before serving

10) RICH BREAKFAST PECAN AND PEAR FARRO

Preparation Time: 20 minutes **Servings:** 4

Ingredients:
- 2 cups water
- ½ tsp salt
- 1 cup farro
- 1 tbsp plant butter
- 2 pears, peeled, cored, and chopped
- ¼ cup chopped pecans

Directions:
- Bring water to a boil in a pot over high heat. Stir in salt and farro. Lower the heat, cover, and simmer for 15 minutes until the farro is tender and the liquid has absorbed. Turn the heat off and add in the butter, pears, and pecans. Cover and rest for 12-15 minutes.
- Serve immediately

11) SIMPLE BLACKBERRY WAFFLES

Preparation Time: 15 minutes **Servings:** 4

Ingredients:
- 1 ½ cups whole-heat flour
- ½ cup old-fashioned oats
- ¼ cup date sugar
- 3 tsp baking powder
- ½ tsp salt
- 1 tsp ground cinnamon
- 2 cups soy milk
- 1 tbsp fresh lemon juice
- 1 tsp lemon zest
- ¼ cup plant butter, melted
- ½ cup fresh blackberries

Directions:
- Preheat the waffle iron.
- In a bowl, mix flour, oats, sugar, baking powder, salt, and cinnamon. Set aside. In another bowl, combine milk, lemon juice, lemon zest, and butter. Pour into the wet ingredients and whisk to combine. Add the batter to the hot greased waffle iron, using approximately a ladleful for each waffle. Cook for 3-5 minutes, until golden brown. Repeat the process until no batter is left.
- Serve topped with blackberries

12) AUTHENTIC WALNUT WAFFLES WITH MAPLE SYRUP

Preparation Time: 15 minutes **Servings:** 4

Ingredients:
- 1 ¾ cups whole-wheat flour
- ⅓ cup coarsely ground walnuts
- 1 tbsp baking powder
- 1 ½p cups soy milk
- 3 tbsp pure maple syrup
- 3 tbsp plant butter, melted

Directions:
- Preheat the waffle iron and grease with oil. Combine the flour, walnuts, baking powder, and salt in a bowl. Set aside. In another bowl, mix the milk and butter. Pour into the walnut mixture and whisk until well combined. Spoon a ladleful of the batter onto the waffle iron.
- Cook for 3-5 minutes, until golden brown. Repeat the process until no batter is left. Top with maple syrup to serve

13) SIMPLE ORANGE AND BRAN CUPS WITH DATES

Preparation Time: 30 minutes **Servings:** 12

Ingredients:
- 1 tsp vegetable oil
- 3 cups bran flakes cereal
- 1 ½ cups whole-wheat flour
- ½ cup dates, chopped
- 3 tsp baking powder
- ½ tsp ground cinnamon
- ½ tsp salt
- ⅓ cup brown sugar
- ¾ cup fresh orange juice

Directions:
- Preheat oven to 400 F. Grease a 12-cup muffin tin with oil.
- Mix the bran flakes, flour, dates, baking powder, cinnamon, and salt in a bowl. In another bowl, combine the sugar and orange juice until blended. Pour into the dry mixture and whisk. Divide the mixture between the cups of the muffin tin. Bake for 20 minutes or until golden brown and set. Cool for a few minutes before removing from the tin and serve

14) EXOTIC MACADAMIA NUTS AND APPLE-DATE COUSCOUS

Preparation Time: 20 minutes **Servings:** 4

Ingredients:
- 3 cups apple juice
- 1 ½ cups couscous
- 1 tsp ground cinnamon
- ¼ tsp ground cloves
- ½ cup dried dates
- ½ cup chopped macadamia nuts

Directions:
- Pour the apple juice into a pot over medium heat and bring to a boil. Stir in couscous, cinnamon, and cloves. Turn the heat off and cover. Let sit for 5 minutes until the liquid is absorbed.
- Using a fork, fluff the couscous and add the dates and macadamia nuts, stir to combine. Serve warm

15) TASTY BLUEBERRY COCONUT MUFFINS

Preparation Time: 30 minutes   **Servings:** 12

Ingredients:

- 1 tbsp coconut oil melted
- 1 cup quick-cooking oats
- 1 cup boiling water
- ½ cup almond milk
- ¼ cup ground flaxseed
- 1 tsp almond extract
- 1 tsp apple cider vinegar
- 1 ½ cups whole-wheat flour
- ½ cup pure date sugar
- 2 tsp baking soda
- A pinch of salt
- 1 cup blueberries

Directions:

- Preheat oven to 400 F.
- In a bowl, stir in the oats with boiling water until they are softened. Pour in the coconut oil, milk, flaxseed, almond extract, and vinegar. Add in the flour, sugar, baking soda, and salt. Gently stir in blueberries.
- Divide the batter between a greased with coconut oil muffin tin. Bake for 20 minutes until lightly brown. Allow cooling for 10 minutes. Using a spatula, run the sides of the muffins to take out. Serve

16) SWISS-STYLE CHARD SCRAMBLED TOFU

Preparation Time: 35 minutes   **Servings:** 5

Ingredients:

- 1 (14-oz) package tofu, crumbled
- 2 tsp olive oil
- 1 onion, chopped
- 3 cloves minced garlic
- 1 celery stalk, chopped
- 2 large carrots, chopped
- 1 tsp chili powder
- ½ tsp ground cumin
- ½ tsp ground turmeric
- Salt and black pepper to taste
- 5 cups Swiss chard

Directions:

- Heat the oil in a skillet over medium heat. Add in the onion, garlic, celery, and carrots. Sauté for 5 minutes. Stir in tofu, chili powder, cumin, turmeric, salt, and pepper, cook for 7-8 minutes more.
- Mix in the Swiss chard and cook until wilted, about 3 minutes. Allow cooling and seal and serve

17) BEST BAKED SPICY EGGPLANT

Preparation Time: 30 minutes   **Servings:** 4

Ingredients:

- 2 large eggplants
- Salt and black pepper to taste
- 2 tbsp plant butter
- 1 tsp red chili flakes
- 4 oz raw ground almonds

- Preheat oven to 400 F.
- Cut off the head of the eggplants and slice the body into 2-inch rounds. Season with salt and black pepper and arrange on a parchment paper-lined baking sheet.
- Drop thin slices of the plant butter on each eggplant slice, sprinkle with red chili flakes, and bake in the oven for 20 minutes.
- Slide the baking sheet out and sprinkle with the almonds. Roast further for 5 minutes or until golden brown. Dish the eggplants and serve with arugula salad

18) VERY GOOD MASHED BROCCOLI WITH ROASTED GARLIC

Preparation Time: 45 minutes   **Servings:** 4

Ingredients:

- ½ head garlic
- 2 tbsp olive oil + for garnish
- 1 head broccoli, cut into florets
- 1 tsp salt
- 4 oz plant butter
- ¼ tsp dried thyme
- Juice and zest of half a lemon
- 4 tbsp coconut cream

Directions:

- Preheat oven to 400 F.
- Use a knife to cut a ¼ inch off the top of the garlic cloves, drizzle with olive oil, and wrap in aluminum foil. Place on a baking sheet and roast for 30 minutes. Remove and set aside when ready.
- Pour the broccoli into a pot, add 3 cups of water, and 1 tsp of salt. Bring to a boil until tender, about 7 minutes. Drain and transfer the broccoli to a bowl. Add the plant butter, thyme, lemon juice and zest, coconut cream, and olive oil. Use an immersion blender to puree the ingredients until smooth and nice. Spoon the mash into serving bowls and garnish with some olive oil. Serve

19) SIMPLE SPICY PISTACHIO DIP

Preparation Time: 10 minutes | **Servings:** 4

Ingredients:
- 3 oz toasted pistachios + for garnish
- 3 tbsp coconut cream
- ¼ cup water
- Juice of half a lemon
- ½ tsp smoked paprika
- Cayenne pepper to taste
- ½ tsp salt
- ½ cup olive oil

Directions:
- Pour the pistachios, coconut cream, water, lemon juice, paprika, cayenne pepper, and salt. Puree the ingredients at high speed until smooth. Add the olive oil and puree a little further. Manage the consistency of the dip by adding more oil or water. Spoon the dip into little bowls, garnish with some pistachios, and serve with julienned celery and carrots

20) HUNGARIAN PAPRIKA ROASTED NUTS

Preparation Time: 10 minutes | **Servings:** 4

Ingredients:
- 8 oz walnuts and pecans
- 1 tsp salt
- 1 tbsp coconut oil
- 1 tsp cumin powder
- 1 tsp paprika powder

- In a bowl, mix walnuts, pecans, salt, coconut oil, cumin powder, and paprika powder until the nuts are well coated with spice and oil. Pour the mixture into a pan and toast while stirring continually. Once the nuts are fragrant and brown, transfer to a bowl. Allow cooling and serve with a chilled berry juice

21) EASY MIXED VEGETABLES WITH BASIL

Preparation Time: 40 minutes | **Servings:** 4

Ingredients:
- 2 medium zucchinis, chopped
- 2 medium yellow squash, chopped
- 1 red onion, cut into 1-inch wedges
- 1 red bell pepper, diced
- 1 cup cherry tomatoes, halved
- 4 tbsp olive oil
- Salt and black pepper to taste
- 3 garlic cloves, minced
- 2/3 cup whole-wheat breadcrumbs
- 1 lemon, zested
- ¼ cup chopped fresh basil

- Preheat the oven to 450 F. Lightly grease a large baking sheet with cooking spray.
- In a medium bowl, add the zucchini, yellow squash, red onion, bell pepper, tomatoes, olive oil, salt, black pepper, and garlic. Toss well and spread the mixture on the baking sheet. Roast in the oven for 25 to 30 minutes or until the vegetables are tender while stirring every 5 minutes.
- Meanwhile, heat the olive oil in a medium skillet and sauté the garlic until fragrant. Mix in the breadcrumbs, lemon zest, and basil. Cook for 2 to 3 minutes. Remove the vegetables from the oven and toss in the breadcrumb's mixture. Serve

22) DELICIOUS ONION RINGS AND KALE DIP

Preparation Time: 35 minutes | **Servings:** 4

Ingredients:
- 1 onion, sliced into rings
- 1 tbsp flaxseed meal + 3 tbsp water
- 1 cup almond flour
- ½ cup grated plant-based Parmesan
- 2 tsp garlic powder
- ½ tbsp sweet paprika powder
- 2 oz chopped kale
- 2 tbsp olive oil
- 2 tbsp dried cilantro
- 1 tbsp dried oregano
- Salt and black pepper to taste
- 1 cup tofu mayonnaise
- 4 tbsp coconut cream
- Juice of ½ a lemon

- Preheat oven to 400 F. In a bowl, mix the flaxseed meal and water and leave the mixture to thicken and fully absorb for 5 minutes. In another bowl, combine almond flour, plant-based Parmesan cheese, half of the garlic powder, sweet paprika, and salt. Line a baking sheet with parchment paper in readiness for the rings. When the vegan "flax egg" is ready, dip in the onion rings one after another, and then into the almond flour mixture. Place the rings on the baking sheet and grease with cooking spray. Bake for 15-20 minutes or until golden brown and crispy. Remove the onion rings into a serving bowl.
- Put kale in a food processor. Add in olive oil, cilantro, oregano, remaining garlic powder, salt, black pepper, tofu mayonnaise, coconut cream, and lemon juice; puree until nice and smooth. Allow the dip to sit for about 10 minutes for the flavors to develop. After, serve the dip with the crispy onion rings

23) PORTUGUESE SOY CHORIZO STUFFED CABBAGE ROLLS

Preparation Time: 35 minutes   **Servings:** 4

Ingredients:
- ¼ cup coconut oil, divided
- 1 large white onion, chopped
- 3 cloves garlic, minced, divided
- 1 cup crumbled soy chorizo
- 1 cup cauliflower rice
- 1 can tomato sauce
- 1 tsp dried oregano
- 1 tsp dried basil
- 8 full green cabbage leaves

Directions:
- Heat half of the coconut oil in a saucepan over medium heat.
- Add half of the onion, half of the garlic, and all of the soy chorizo. Sauté for 5 minutes or until the chorizo has browned further, and the onion softened. Stir in the cauli rice, season with salt and black pepper, and cook for 3 to 4 minutes. Turn the heat off and set the pot aside.
- Heat the remaining oil in a saucepan over medium heat, add, and sauté the remaining onion and garlic until fragrant and soft. Pour in the tomato sauce, and season with salt, black pepper, oregano, and basil. Add ¼ cup water and simmer the sauce for 10 minutes.
- While the sauce cooks, lay the cabbage leaves on a flat surface and spoon the soy chorizo mixture into the middle of each leaf. Roll the leaves to secure the filling. Place the cabbage rolls in the tomato sauce and cook further for 10 minutes. When ready, serve the cabbage rolls with sauce over mashed broccoli or with mixed seed bread

24) TROPICAL BANANA TANGERINE TOAST

Preparation Time: 25 minutes   **Servings:** 4

Ingredients:
- 3 bananas
- 1 cup almond milk
- Zest and juice of 1 tangerine
- 1 tsp ground cinnamon
- ¼ tsp grated nutmeg
- 4 slices bread
- 1 tbsp olive oil

Directions:
- Blend the bananas, almond milk, tangerine juice, tangerine zest, cinnamon, and nutmeg until smooth in a food processor. Spread into a baking dish. Submerge the bread slices in the mixture for 3-4 minutes.
- Heat the oil in a skillet over medium heat. Fry the bread for 5 minutes until golden brown. Serve hot

25) EASY MAPLE BANANA OATS

Preparation Time: 35 minutes   **Servings:** 4

Ingredients:
- 3 cups water
- 1 cup steel-cut oats
- 2 bananas, mashed
- ¼ cup pumpkin seeds
- 2 tbsp maple syrup
- A pinch of salt

Directions:
- Bring water to a boil in a pot, add in oats, and lower the heat. Cook for 20-30 minutes. Put in the mashed bananas, cook for 3-5 minutes more. Stir in maple syrup, pumpkin seeds, and salt. Serve

26) TASTY GINGERBREAD BELGIAN WAFFLES

Preparation Time: 25 minutes

Servings: 3

Ingredients:
- 1 cup all-purpose flour
- 1 tsp baking powder
- 1 tbsp brown sugar
- 1 tsp ground ginger
- 1 cup almond milk
- 1 tsp vanilla extract
- 2 olive oil

Directions:
- Preheat a waffle iron according to the manufacturer's instructions.
- In a mixing bowl, thoroughly combine the flour, baking powder, brown sugar, ground ginger, almond milk, vanilla extract and olive oil.
- Beat until everything is well blended.
- Ladle 1/3 of the batter into the preheated waffle iron and cook until the waffles are golden and crisp. Repeat with the remaining batter.
- Serve your waffles with blackberry jam, if desired. Enjoy

27) EASY BANANA AND WALNUTS PORRIDGE

Preparation Time: 15 minutes

Servings: 4

Ingredients:
- 1 cup rolled oats
- 1 cup spelt flakes
- 2 cups unsweetened almond milk
- 4 tbsp agave nectar
- 4 tbsp walnuts, chopped
- 2 bananas, sliced

Directions:
- In a nonstick skillet, fry the oats and spelt flakes until fragrant, working in batches.
- Bring the milk to a boil and add in the oats, spelt flakes and agave nectar.
- Turn the heat to a simmer and let it cook for 6 to 7 minutes, stirring occasionally. Top with walnuts and bananas and serve warm. Enjoy

Chapter 2. LUNCH

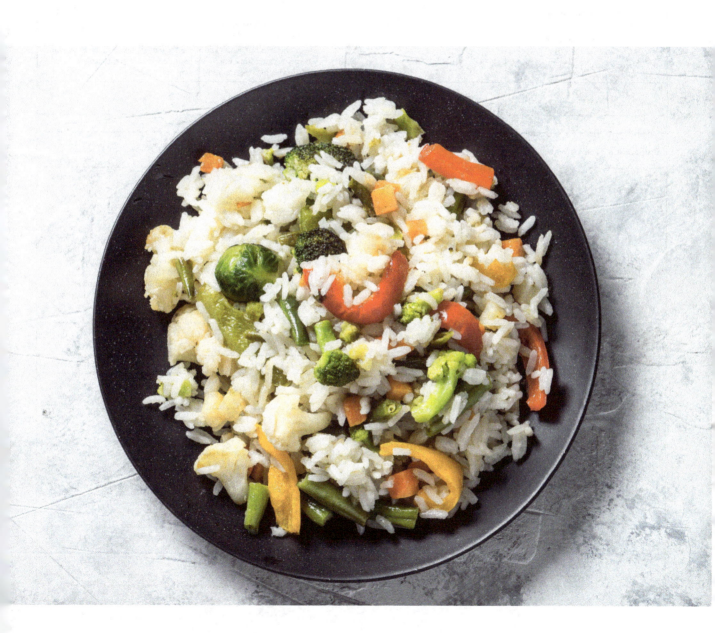

28) ITALIAN MUSHROOM SOUP OF MEDLEY

Preparation Time: 40 minutes

Servings: 4

Ingredients:
- 4 oz unsalted plant butter
- 1 small onion, finely chopped
- 1 clove garlic, minced
- 5 oz button mushrooms, chopped
- 5 oz cremini mushrooms, chopped
- 5 oz shiitake mushrooms, chopped
- ½ lb celery root, chopped
- ½ tsp dried rosemary
- 1 vegetable stock cube, crushed
- 1 tbsp plain vinegar
- 1 cup coconut cream
- 4 – 6 leaves basil, chopped

Directions:
- Place a saucepan over medium-high heat, add the plant butter to melt, then sauté the onion, garlic, mushrooms, and celery root in the butter until golden brown and fragrant, about 6 minutes. Fetch out some mushrooms and reserve for garnishing. Add the rosemary, 3 cups of water, stock cube, and vinegar. Stir the mixture and bring it to a boil for 6 minutes. After, reduce the heat and simmer the soup for 15 minutes or until the celery is soft.
- Mix in the coconut cream and puree the ingredients using an immersion blender. Simmer for 2 minutes. Spoon the soup into serving bowls, garnish with the reserved mushrooms and basil. Serve

29) MEDITERRANEAN DILL CAULIFLOWER SOUP

Preparation Time: 26 minutes

Servings: 4

Ingredients:
- 2 tbsp coconut oil
- ½ lb celery root, trimmed
- 1 garlic clove
- 1 medium white onion
- ¼ cup fresh dill, roughly chopped
- 1 tsp cumin powder
- ¼ tsp nutmeg powder
- 1 head cauliflower, cut into florets
- 3 ½ cups seasoned vegetable stock
- 5 oz plant butter
- Juice from 1 lemon
- ¼ cup coconut whipping cream

Directions:
- Set a pot over medium heat, add the coconut oil and allow heating until no longer shimmering.
- Add the celery root, garlic clove, and onion; sauté the vegetables until fragrant and soft, about 5 minutes. Stir in the dill, cumin, and nutmeg, and fry further for 1 minute. Mix in the cauliflower florets and vegetable stock. Bring the soup to a boil for 12 to 15 minutes or until the cauliflower is soft. Turn the heat off. Add the plant butter and lemon juice. Puree the ingredients with an immersion blender until smooth. Mix in coconut whipping cream and season the soup with salt and black pepper. Serve warm

30) SPECIAL FENNEL BROCCOLI SOUP

Preparation Time: 25 minutes

Servings: 4

Ingredients:
- 1 fennel bulb, chopped
- 10 oz broccoli, cut into florets
- 3 cups vegetable stock
- Salt and black pepper to taste
- 1 garlic clove
- 1 cup cashew cream cheese
- 3 oz plant butter
- ½ cup chopped fresh oregano

Directions:
- Put the fennel and broccoli into a pot, and cover with the vegetable stock. Bring the ingredients to a boil over medium heat until the vegetables are soft, about 10 minutes. Season the liquid with salt and black pepper, and drop in the garlic. Simmer the soup for 5 to 7 minutes and turn the heat off.
- Pour the cream cheese, plant butter, and oregano into the soup; puree the ingredients with an immersion blender until completely smooth. Adjust the taste with salt and black pepper. Spoon the soup into serving bowls and serve

31) EASY BEAN SOUP ASIAN-STYLE

Preparation Time: 55 minutes | | **Servings:** 4

Ingredients:
- 1 cup canned cannellini beans
- 2 tsp curry powder
- 2 tsp olive oil
- 1 red onion, diced
- 1 tbsp minced fresh ginger
- 2 cubed sweet potatoes
- 1 cup sliced zucchini
- Salt and black pepper to taste
- 4 cups vegetable stock
- 1 bunch spinach, chopped
- Toasted sesame seeds

Directions:
- Mix the beans with 1 tsp of curry powder until well combined. Warm the oil in a pot over medium heat. Place the onion and ginger and cook for 5 minutes until soft. Add in sweet potatoes and cook for 10 minutes. Put in zucchini and cook for 5 minutes. Season with the remaining curry, pepper, and salt.
- Pour in the stock and bring to a boil. Lower the heat and simmer for 25 minutes. Stir in beans and spinach. Cook until the spinach wilts and remove from the heat. Garnish with sesame seeds to serve

32) TORTILLA MEXICAN-STYLE SOUP

Preparation Time: 40 minutes | | **Servings:** 4

Ingredients:
- 1 (14.5-oz) can diced tomatoes
- 1 (4-oz) can green chiles, chopped
- 2 tbsp olive oil
- 1 cup canned sweet corn
- 1 red onion, chopped
- 2 garlic cloves, minced
- 2 jalapeño peppers, sliced
- 4 cups vegetable broth
- 8 oz seitan, cut into ¼-inch strips
- Salt and black pepper to taste
- ¼ cup chopped fresh cilantro
- 3 tbsp fresh lime juice
- 4 corn tortillas, cut into strips
- 1 ripe avocado, chopped

Directions:
- Preheat oven to 350 F. Heat the oil in a pot over medium heat. Place sweet corn, garlic, jalapeño, and onion and cook for 5 minutes. Stir in broth, seitan, tomatoes, canned chiles, salt, and pepper. Bring to a boil, then lower the heat and simmer for 20 minutes. Put in the cilantro and lime juice, stir. Adjust the seasoning.
- Meanwhile, arrange the tortilla strips on a baking sheet and bake for 8 minutes until crisp. Serve the soup into bowls and top with tortilla strips and avocado

33) HOT BEAN SPICY SOUP

Preparation Time: 40 minutes | | **Servings:** 4

Ingredients:
- 2 tbsp olive oil
- 1 medium onion, chopped
- 2 large garlic cloves, minced
- 1 carrot, chopped
- 1 (15.5-oz) can cannellini beans, drained
- 5 cups vegetable broth
- ¼ tsp crushed red pepper
- Salt and black pepper to taste
- 3 cups chopped baby spinach

Directions:
- Heat oil in a pot over medium heat. Place in carrot, onion, and garlic and cook for 3 minutes. Put in beans, broth, red pepper, salt, and black pepper and stir. Bring to a boil, then lower the heat and simmer for 25 minutes. Stir in baby spinach and cook for 5 minutes until the spinach wilts. Serve warm

34) SPECIAL MUSHROOM RICE WINE SOUP

Preparation Time: 25 minutes | | **Servings:** 4

Ingredients:
- 2 tbsp olive oil
- 4 green onions, chopped
- 1 carrot, chopped
- 8 oz shiitake mushrooms, sliced
- 3 tbsp rice wine
- 2 tbsp soy sauce
- 4 cups vegetable broth
- Salt and black pepper to taste
- 2 tbsp parsley, chopped

Directions:
- Heat the oil in a pot over medium heat. Place the green onions and carrot and cook for 5 minutes.
- Stir in mushrooms, rice wine, soy sauce, broth, salt, and pepper. Bring to a boil, then lower the heat and simmer for 15 minutes. Top with parsley and serve warm

35) TASTY BEAN TANGY TOMATO SOUP

Preparation Time: 30 minutes **Servings:** 5

Ingredients:
- 2 tsp olive oil
- 1 onion, chopped
- 2 garlic cloves, minced
- 1 cup mushrooms, chopped
- Sea salt to taste
- 1 tbsp dried basil
- ½ tbsp dried oregano
- 1 (19-oz) can diced tomatoes
- 1 (14-oz) can kidney beans, drained
- 5 cups water
- 2 cups chopped mustard greens

Directions:
- Heat the oil in a pot over medium heat. Place in the onion, garlic, mushrooms, and salt and cook for 5 minutes. Stir in basil and oregano, tomatoes, and beans. Pour in water and stir. Simmer for 20 minutes and add in mustard greens; cook for 5 minutes until greens soften. Serve immediately

36) EASY SPINACH AND POTATO SOUP

Preparation Time: 55 minutes **Servings:** 4

Ingredients:
- 2 tbsp olive oil
- 1 onion, chopped
- 2 garlic cloves, minced
- 4 cups vegetable broth
- 2 russet potatoes, cubed
- ½ tsp dried oregano
- ¼ tsp crushed red pepper
- 1 bay leaf
- Salt to taste
- 4 cups chopped spinach
- 1 cup green lentils, rinsed

Directions:
- Warm the oil in a pot over medium heat. Place the onion and garlic and cook covered for 5 minutes. Stir in broth, potatoes, oregano, red pepper, bay leaf, lentils, and salt. Bring to a boil, then lower the heat and simmer uncovered for 30 minutes. Add in spinach and cook for another 5 minutes. Discard the bay leaf and serve immediately

37) MEXICAN BEAN TURMERIC SOUP

Preparation Time: 50 minutes **Servings:** 6

Ingredients:
- 3 tbsp olive oil
- 1 onion, chopped
- 2 carrots, chopped
- 1 sweet potato, chopped
- 1 yellow bell pepper, chopped
- 2 garlic cloves, minced
- 4 tomatoes, chopped
- 6 cups vegetable broth
- 1 bay leaf
- Salt to taste
- 1 tsp ground cayenne pepper
- 1 (15.5-oz) can white beans, drained
- ⅓ cup whole-wheat pasta
- ¼ tsp turmeric

Directions:
- Heat the oil in a pot over medium heat. Place onion, carrots, sweet potato, bell pepper, and garlic. Cook for 5 minutes. Add in tomatoes, broth, bay leaf, salt, and cayenne pepper. Stir and bring to a boil. Lower the heat and simmer for 10 minutes. Put in white beans and simmer for 15 more minutes.
- Cook the pasta in a pot with boiling salted water and turmeric for 8-10 minutes, until pasta is al dente. Strain and transfer to the soup. Discard the bay leaf. Spoon into a bowl and serve

38) TROPICAL COCONUT ARUGULA SOUP

Preparation Time: 30 minutes **Servings:** 4

Ingredients:
- 1 tsp coconut oil
- 1 onion, diced
- 2 cups green beans
- 4 cups water
- 1 cup arugula, chopped
- 1 tbsp fresh mint, chopped
- Sea salt and black pepper to taste
- ¾ cup coconut milk

Directions:
- Place a pot over medium heat and heat the coconut oil. Add in the onion and sauté for 5 minutes. Pour in green beans and water. Bring to a boil, lower the heat and stir in arugula, mint, salt, and pepper. Simmer for 10 minutes. Stir in coconut milk. Transfer to a food processor and blitz the soup until smooth. Serve

39) AUTHENTIC LENTIL SOUP WITH SWISS CHARD

Preparation Time: 25 minutes **Servings:** 5

Ingredients:
- 2 tbsp olive oil
- 1 white onion, chopped
- 1 tsp garlic, minced
- 2 large carrots, chopped
- 1 parsnip, chopped
- 2 stalks celery, chopped
- 2 bay leaves
- 1/2 tsp dried thyme
- 1/4 tsp ground cumin
- 5 cups roasted vegetable broth
- 1 ¼ cups brown lentils, soaked overnight and rinsed
- 2 cups Swiss chard, torn into pieces

Directions:
- In a heavy-bottomed pot, heat the olive oil over a moderate heat. Now, sauté the vegetables along with the spices for about 3 minutes until they are just tender.
- Add in the vegetable broth and lentils, bringing it to a boil. Immediately turn the heat to a simmer and add in the bay leaves. Let it cook for about 15 minutes or until lentils are tender.
- Add in the Swiss chard, cover and let it simmer for 5 minutes more or until the chard wilts.
- Serve in individual bowls and enjoy

40) AUTUMN SPICY FARRO SOUP

Preparation Time: 30 minutes **Servings:** 4

Ingredients:
- 2 tbsp olive oil
- 1 medium-sized leek, chopped
- 1 medium-sized turnip, sliced
- 2 Italian peppers, seeded and chopped
- 1 jalapeno pepper, minced
- 2 potatoes, peeled and diced
- 4 cups vegetable broth
- 1 cup farro, rinsed
- 1/2 tsp granulated garlic
- 1/2 tsp turmeric powder
- 1 bay laurel
- 2 cups spinach, turn into pieces

Directions:
- In a heavy-bottomed pot, heat the olive oil over a moderate heat. Now, sauté the leek, turnip, peppers and potatoes for about 5 minutes until they are crisp-tender.
- Add in the vegetable broth, farro, granulated garlic, turmeric and bay laurel; bring it to a boil.
- Immediately turn the heat to a simmer. Let it cook for about 25 minutes or until farro and potatoes have softened.
- Add in the spinach and remove the pot from the heat; let the spinach sit in the residual heat until it wilts. Enjoy

41) ALL COLORED CHICKPEA SALAD

Preparation Time: 30 minutes

Servings: 4

Ingredients:
- 16 ounces canned chickpeas, drained
- 1 medium avocado, sliced
- 1 bell pepper, seeded and sliced
- 1 large tomato, sliced
- 2 cucumber, diced
- 1 red onion, sliced
- 1/2 tsp garlic, minced
- 1/4 cup fresh parsley, chopped
- 1/4 cup olive oil
- 2 tbsp apple cider vinegar
- 1/2 lime, freshly squeezed
- Sea salt and ground black pepper, to taste

Directions:
- Toss all the ingredients in a salad bowl.
- Place the salad in your refrigerator for about 1 hour before serving.
- Enjoy

42) MEDITERRANEAN-STYLE LENTIL SALAD

Preparation Time: 20 minutes + chilling time

Servings: 5

Ingredients:
- 1 ½ cups red lentil, rinsed
- 1 tsp deli mustard
- 1/2 lemon, freshly squeezed
- 2 tbsp tamari sauce
- 2 scallion stalks, chopped
- 1/4 cup extra-virgin olive oil
- 2 garlic cloves, minced
- 1 cup butterhead lettuce, torn into pieces
- 2 tbsp fresh parsley, chopped
- 2 tbsp fresh cilantro, chopped
- 1 tsp fresh basil
- 1 tsp fresh oregano
- 1 ½ cups cherry tomatoes, halved
- 3 ounces Kalamata olives, pitted and halved

Directions:
- In a large-sized saucepan, bring 4 ½ cups of the water and the red lentils to a boil.
- Immediately turn the heat to a simmer and continue to cook your lentils for about 15 minutes or until tender. Drain and let it cool completely.
- Transfer the lentils to a salad bowl; toss the lentils with the remaining ingredients until well combined.
- Serve chilled or at room temperature. Enjoy

43) DELICIOUS ROASTED AVOCADO AND ASPARAGUS SALAD

Preparation Time: 20 minutes + chilling time

Servings: 4

Ingredients:
- 1 pound asparagus, trimmed, cut into bite-sized pieces
- 1 white onion, chopped
- 2 garlic cloves, minced
- 1 Roma tomato, sliced
- 1/4 cup olive oil
- 1/4 cup balsamic vinegar
- 1 tbsp stone-ground mustard
- 2 tbsp fresh parsley, chopped
- 1 tbsp fresh cilantro, chopped
- 1 tbsp fresh basil, chopped
- Sea salt and ground black pepper, to taste
- 1 small avocado, pitted and diced
- 1/2 cup pine nuts, roughly chopped

Directions:
- Begin by preheating your oven to 420 degrees F.
- Toss the asparagus with 1 tbsp of the olive oil and arrange them on a parchment-lined roasting pan.
- Bake for about 15 minutes, rotating the pan once or twice to promote even cooking. Let it cool completely and place in your salad bowl.
- Toss the asparagus with the vegetables, olive oil, vinegar, mustard and herbs. Salt and pepper to taste.
- Toss to combine and top with avocado and pine nuts. Enjoy

44) SPECIAL GREEN BEAN CREAM SALAD WITH PINE NUTS

Preparation Time: 10 minutes + chilling time

Servings: 5

Ingredients:
- 1 ½ pounds green beans, trimmed
- 2 medium tomatoes, diced
- 2 bell peppers, seeded and diced
- 4 tbsp shallots, chopped
- 1/2 cup pine nuts, roughly chopped
- 1/2 cup vegan mayonnaise
- 1 tbsp deli mustard
- 2 tbsp fresh basil, chopped
- 2 tbsp fresh parsley, chopped
- 1/2 tsp red pepper flakes, crushed
- Sea salt and freshly ground black pepper, to taste

Directions:
- Boil the green beans in a large saucepan of salted water until they are just tender or about 2 minutes.
- Drain and let the beans cool completely; then, transfer them to a salad bowl. Toss the beans with the remaining ingredients.
- Taste and adjust the seasonings. Enjoy

---

45) EASY KALE CANNELLINI BEAN SOUP

Preparation Time: 25 minutes

Servings: 5

Ingredients:
- 1 tbsp olive oil
- 1/2 tsp ginger, minced
- 1/2 tsp cumin seeds
- 1 red onion, chopped
- 1 carrot, trimmed and chopped
- 1 parsnip, trimmed and chopped
- 2 garlic cloves, minced
- 5 cups vegetable broth
- 12 ounces Cannellini beans, drained
- 2 cups kale, torn into pieces
- Sea salt and ground black pepper, to taste

Directions:
- In a heavy-bottomed pot, heat the olive over medium-high heat. Now, sauté the ginger and cumin for 1 minute or so.
- Now, add in the onion, carrot and parsnip; continue sautéing an additional 3 minutes or until the vegetables are just tender.
- Add in the garlic and continue to sauté for 1 minute or until aromatic.
- Then, pour in the vegetable broth and bring to a boil. Immediately reduce the heat to a simmer and let it cook for 10 minutes.
- Fold in the Cannellini beans and kale; continue to simmer until the kale wilts and everything is thoroughly heated. Season with salt and pepper to taste.
- Ladle into individual bowls and serve hot. Enjoy

---

46) DELICIOUS MUSHROOM SOUP WITH HEARTY CREAM

Preparation Time: 15 minutes

Servings: 5

Ingredients:
- 2 tbsp soy butter
- 1 large shallot, chopped
- 20 ounces Cremini mushrooms, sliced
- 2 cloves garlic, minced
- 4 tbsp flaxseed meal
- 5 cups vegetable broth
- 1 1/3 cups full-fat coconut milk
- 1 bay leaf
- Sea salt and ground black pepper, to taste

Directions:
- In a stockpot, melt the vegan butter over medium-high heat. Once hot, cook the shallot for about 3 minutes until tender and fragrant.
- Add in the mushrooms and garlic and continue cooking until the mushrooms have softened. Add in the flaxseed meal and continue to cook for 1 minute or so.
- Add in the remaining ingredients. Let it simmer, covered and continue to cook for 5 to 6 minutes more until your soup has thickened slightly.
- Enjoy

47) ITALIAN-STYLE AUTHENTIC PANZANELLA SALAD

Preparation Time: 35 minutes

Servings: 3

Ingredients:
- 3 cups artisan bread, broken into 1-inch cubes
- 3/4-pound asparagus, trimmed and cut into bite-sized pieces
- 4 tbsp extra-virgin olive oil
- 1 red onion, chopped
- 2 tbsp fresh lime juice
- 1 tsp deli mustard
- 2 medium heirloom tomatoes, diced
- 2 cups arugula
- 2 cups baby spinach
- 2 Italian peppers, seeded and sliced
- Sea salt and ground black pepper, to taste

Directions:
- Arrange the bread cubes on a parchment-lined baking sheet. Bake in the preheated oven at 310 degrees F for about 20 minutes, rotating the baking sheet twice during the baking time; reserve.
- Turn the oven to 420 degrees F and toss the asparagus with 1 tbsp of olive oil. Roast the asparagus for about 15 minutes or until crisp-tender.
- Toss the remaining ingredients in a salad bowl; top with the roasted asparagus and toasted bread.
- Enjoy

48) ASIAN BLACK BEAN QUINOA SALAD

Preparation Time: 15 minutes + chilling time

Servings: 4

Ingredients:
- 2 cups water
- 1 cup quinoa, rinsed
- 16 ounces canned black beans, drained
- 2 Roma tomatoes, sliced
- 1 red onion, thinly sliced
- 1 cucumber, seeded and chopped
- 2 cloves garlic, pressed or minced
- 2 Italian peppers, seeded and sliced
- 2 tbsp fresh parsley, chopped
- 2 tbsp fresh cilantro, chopped
- 1/4 cup olive oil
- 1 lemon, freshly squeezed
- 1 tbsp apple cider vinegar
- 1/2 tsp dried dill weed
- 1/2 tsp dried oregano
- Sea salt and ground black pepper, to taste

Directions:
- Place the water and quinoa in a saucepan and bring it to a rolling boil. Immediately turn the heat to a simmer.
- Let it simmer for about 13 minutes until the quinoa has absorbed all of the water; fluff the quinoa with a fork and let it cool completely. Then, transfer the quinoa to a salad bowl.
- Add the remaining ingredients to the salad bowl and toss to combine well. Enjoy

49) MOROCCAN POWER BULGUR SALAD WITH HERBS

Preparation Time: 20 minutes + chilling time

Servings: 4

Ingredients:
- 2 cups water
- 1 cup bulgur
- 12 ounces canned chickpeas, drained
- 1 Persian cucumber, thinly sliced
- 2 bell peppers, seeded and thinly sliced
- 1 jalapeno pepper, seeded and thinly sliced
- 2 Roma tomatoes, sliced
- 1 onion, thinly sliced
- 2 tbsp fresh basil, chopped
- 2 tbsp fresh parsley, chopped
- 2 tbsp fresh mint, chopped
- 2 tbsp fresh chives, chopped
- 4 tbsp olive oil
- 1 tbsp balsamic vinegar
- 1 tbsp lemon juice
- 1 tsp fresh garlic, pressed
- Sea salt and freshly ground black pepper, to taste
- 2 tbsp nutritional yeast
- 1/2 cup Kalamata olives, sliced

Directions:
- In a saucepan, bring the water and bulgur to a boil. Immediately turn the heat to a simmer and let it cook for about 20 minutes or until the bulgur is tender and water is almost absorbed. Fluff with a fork and spread on a large tray to let cool.
- Place the bulgur in a salad bowl followed by the chickpeas, cucumber, peppers, tomatoes, onion, basil, parsley, mint and chives.
- In a small mixing dish, whisk the olive oil, balsamic vinegar, lemon juice, garlic, salt and black pepper. Dress the salad and toss to combine.
- Sprinkle nutritional yeast over the top, garnish with olives and serve at room temperature. Enjoy

50) AUTHENTIC ROASTED PEPPER SALAD

Preparation Time: 15 minutes + chilling time **Servings:** 3

Ingredients:
- 6 bell peppers
- 3 tbsp extra-virgin olive oil
- 3 tsp red wine vinegar
- 3 garlic cloves, finely chopped
- 2 tbsp fresh parsley, chopped
- Sea salt and freshly cracked black pepper, to taste
- 1/2 tsp red pepper flakes
- 6 tbsp pine nuts, roughly chopped

Directions:
- Broil the peppers on a parchment-lined baking sheet for about 10 minutes, rotating the pan halfway through the cooking time, until they are charred on all sides.
- Then, cover the peppers with a plastic wrap to steam. Discard the skin, seeds and cores.
- Slice the peppers into strips and toss them with the remaining ingredients. Place in your refrigerator until ready to serve. Enjoy

51) AUTUMN HEARTY QUINOA SOUP

Preparation Time: 25 minutes **Servings:** 4

Ingredients:
- 2 tbsp olive oil
- 1 onion, chopped
- 2 carrots, peeled and chopped
- 1 parsnip, chopped
- 1 celery stalk, chopped
- 1 cup yellow squash, chopped
- 4 garlic cloves, pressed or minced
- 4 cups roasted vegetable broth
- 2 medium tomatoes, crushed
- 1 cup quinoa
- Sea salt and ground black pepper, to taste
- 1 bay laurel
- 2 cup Swiss chard, tough ribs removed and torn into pieces
- 2 tbsp Italian parsley, chopped

Directions:
- In a heavy-bottomed pot, heat the olive over medium-high heat. Now, sauté the onion, carrot, parsnip, celery and yellow squash for about 3 minutes or until the vegetables are just tender.
- Add in the garlic and continue to sauté for 1 minute or until aromatic.
- Then, stir in the vegetable broth, tomatoes, quinoa, salt, pepper and bay laurel; bring to a boil. Immediately reduce the heat to a simmer and let it cook for 13 minutes.
- Fold in the Swiss chard; continue to simmer until the chard wilts.
- Ladle into individual bowls and serve garnished with the fresh parsley. Enjoy

52) SPECIAL GREEN LENTIL SALAD

Preparation Time: 20 minutes + chilling time **Servings:** 5

Ingredients:
- 1 ½ cups green lentils, rinsed
- 2 cups arugula
- 2 cups Romaine lettuce, torn into pieces
- 1 cup baby spinach
- 1/4 cup fresh basil, chopped
- 1/2 cup shallots, chopped
- 2 garlic cloves, finely chopped
- 1/4 cup oil-packed sun-dried tomatoes, rinsed and chopped
- 5 tbsp extra-virgin olive oil
- 3 tbsp fresh lemon juice
- Sea salt and ground black pepper, to taste

Directions:
- In a large-sized saucepan, bring 4 ½ cups of the water and red lentils to a boil.
- Immediately turn the heat to a simmer and continue to cook your lentils for a further 15 to 17 minutes or until they've softened but not mushy. Drain and let it cool completely.
- Transfer the lentils to a salad bowl; toss the lentils with the remaining ingredients until well combined.
- Serve chilled or at room temperature. Enjoy

53) EASY CHICKPEA, ACORN SQUASH, AND COUSCOUS SOUP

Preparation Time: 20 minutes   **Servings:** 4

Ingredients:
- 2 tbsp olive oil
- 1 shallot, chopped
- 1 carrot, trimmed and chopped
- 2 cups acorn squash, chopped
- 1 stalk celery, chopped
- 1 tsp garlic, finely chopped
- 1 tsp dried rosemary, chopped
- 1 tsp dried thyme, chopped
- 2 cups cream of onion soup
- 2 cups water
- 1 cup dry couscous
- Sea salt and ground black pepper, to taste
- 1/2 tsp red pepper flakes
- 6 ounces canned chickpeas, drained
- 2 tbsp fresh lemon juice

Directions:
- In a heavy-bottomed pot, heat the olive over medium-high heat. Now, sauté the shallot, carrot, acorn squash and celery for about 3 minutes or until the vegetables are just tender.
- Add in the garlic, rosemary and thyme and continue to sauté for 1 minute or until aromatic.
- Then, stir in the soup, water, couscous, salt, black pepper and red pepper flakes; bring to a boil. Immediately reduce the heat to a simmer and let it cook for 12 minutes.
- Fold in the canned chickpeas; continue to simmer until heated through or about 5 minutes more.
- Ladle into individual bowls and drizzle with the lemon juice over the top. Enjoy

54) SPECIAL PUMPKIN CAYENNE SOUP

Preparation Time: 55 minutes   **Servings:** 6

Ingredients:
- 1 (2-pound) pumpkin, sliced
- 3 tbsp olive oil
- 1 tsp salt
- 2 red bell peppers
- 1 onion, halved
- 1 head garlic
- 6 cups water
- Zest and juice of 1 lime
- ¼ tsp cayenne pepper
- ½ tsp ground coriander
- ½ tsp ground cumin
- Toasted pumpkin seeds

Directions:
- Preheat oven to 350 F.
- Brush the pumpkin slices with oil and sprinkle with salt. Arrange the slices skin-side-down and on a greased baking dish and bake for 20 minutes. Brush the onion with oil. Cut the top of the garlic head and brush with oil.
- When the pumpkin is ready, add in bell peppers, onion, and garlic, and bake for another 10 minutes. Allow cooling.
- Take out the flesh from the pumpkin skin and transfer to a food processor. Cut the pepper roughly, peel and cut the onion, and remove the cloves from the garlic head. Transfer to the food processor and pour in the water, lime zest, and lime juice.
- Blend the soup until smooth. If it's very thick, add a bit of water to reach your desired consistency. Sprinkle with salt, cayenne, coriander, and cumin. Serve

55) EASY ZUCCHINI CREAM SOUP WITH WALNUTS

Preparation Time: 45 minutes   **Servings:** 4

Ingredients:
- 3 zucchinis, chopped
- 2 tsp olive oil
- Sea salt and black pepper to taste
- 1 onion, diced
- 4 cups vegetable stock
- 3 tsp ground sage
- 3 tbsp nutritional yeast
- 1 cup non-dairy milk
- ¼ cup toasted walnuts

Directions:
- Heat the oil in a skillet and place zucchini, onion, salt, and pepper; cook for 5 minutes. Pour in vegetable stock and bring to a boil. Lower the heat and simmer for 15 minutes. Stir in sage, nutritional yeast, and milk. Purée the soup with a blender until smooth. Serve garnished with toasted walnuts and pepper

56) TRADITIONAL RAMEN SOUP

Preparation Time: 25 minutes

Servings: 4

Ingredients:
- 7 oz Japanese buckwheat noodles
- 4 tbsp sesame paste
- 1 cup canned pinto beans, drained
- 2 tbsp fresh cilantro, chopped
- 2 scallions, thinly sliced

Directions:
- In boiling salted water, add in the noodles and cook for 5 minutes over low heat. Remove a cup of the noodle water to a bowl and add in the sesame paste; stir until it has dissolved. Pour the sesame mix in the pot with the noodles, add in pinto beans, and stir until everything is hot. Serve topped with cilantro and scallions in individual bowls

57) MEXICAN BLACK-EYED PEA SOUP

Preparation Time: 45 minutes

Servings: 6

Ingredients:
- 2 carrots, chopped
- 1 onion, chopped
- 2 cups canned dried black-eyed peas
- 1 tbsp soy sauce
- 3 tsp dried thyme
- 1 tsp onion powder
- ½ tsp garlic powder
- Salt and black pepper to taste
- ¼ cup chopped pitted black olives

Directions:
- Place carrots, onion, black-eyed peas, 3 cups water, soy sauce, thyme, onion powder, garlic powder, and pepper in a pot. Bring to a boil, then reduce the heat to low. Cook for 20 minutes. Allow cooling for a few minutes. Transfer to a food processor and blend until smooth. Stir in black olives. Serve

58) GREEK LEEKS CAULIFLOWER SOUP

Preparation Time: 25 minutes

Servings: 4

Ingredients:
- 2 tbsp olive oil
- 3 leeks, thinly sliced
- 1 head cauliflower, cut into florets
- 4 cups vegetable stock
- Salt and black pepper to taste
- 3 tbsp chopped fresh chives

Directions:
- Heat the oil in a pot over medium heat. Place the leeks and sauté for 5 minutes. Add in broccoli, vegetable stock, salt, and pepper and cook for 10 minutes. Blend the soup until purée in a food processor. Top with chives and serve

59) ITALIAN LENTIL LIME SOUP

Preparation Time: 35 minutes

Servings: 2

Ingredients:
- 1 tsp olive oil
- 1 onion, chopped
- 6 garlic cloves, minced
- 1 tsp chili powder
- ½ tsp ground cinnamon
- Salt to taste
- 1 cup yellow lentils
- 1 canned crushed tomatoes
- 2 cups water
- 1 celery stalk, chopped
- 2 cups chopped collard greens

Directions:
- Heat oil in a pot over medium heat. Place onion and garlic and cook for 5 minutes. Stir in chili powder, celery, cinnamon, and salt. Pour in lentils, tomatoes and juices, and water. Bring to a boil, then lower the heat and simmer for 15 minutes. Stir in collard greens. Cook for an additional 5 minutes. Serve

60) ASIAN RICE, SPINACH, AND BEAN SOUP

Preparation Time: 45 minutes

Servings: 6

Ingredients:
- 6 cups baby spinach
- 2 tbsp olive oil
- 1 onion, chopped
- 2 garlic cloves, minced
- 1 (15.5-oz) can black-eyed peas
- 6 cups vegetable broth
- Salt and black pepper to taste
- ½ cup brown rice
- Tabasco sauce, for serving

Directions:
- Heat oil in a pot over medium heat. Place the onion and garlic and sauté for 3 minutes. Pour in broth and season with salt and pepper. Bring to a boil, then lower the heat and stir in rice. Simmer for 15 minutes. Stir in peas and spinach and cook for another 5 minutes. Serve topped with Tabasco sauce

61) CREAMY POTATO SOUP WITH HERBS

Preparation Time: 40 minutes

Servings: 4

Ingredients:
- 2 tbsp olive oil
- 1 onion, chopped
- 1 celery stalk, chopped
- 4 large potatoes, peeled and chopped
- 2 garlic cloves, minced
- 1 tsp fresh basil, chopped
- 1 tsp fresh parsley, chopped
- 1 tsp fresh rosemary, chopped
- 1 bay laurel
- 1 tsp ground allspice
- 4 cups vegetable stock
- Salt and fresh ground black pepper, to taste
- 2 tbsp fresh chives chopped

Directions:
- In a heavy-bottomed pot, heat the olive oil over medium-high heat. Once hot, sauté the onion, celery and potatoes for about 5 minutes, stirring periodically.
- Add in the garlic, basil, parsley, rosemary, bay laurel and allspice and continue sautéing for 1 minute or until fragrant.
- Now, add in the vegetable stock, salt and black pepper and bring to a rapid boil. Immediately reduce the heat to a simmer and let it cook for about 30 minutes.
- Puree the soup using an immersion blender until creamy and uniform.
- Reheat your soup and serve with fresh chives. Enjoy

62)

63) ASIAN QUINOA AND AVOCADO SALAD

Preparation Time: 15 minutes + chilling time

Servings: 4

Ingredients:
- 1 cup quinoa, rinsed
- 1 onion, chopped
- 1 tomato, diced
- 2 roasted peppers, cut into strips
- 2 tbsp parsley, chopped
- 2 tbsp basil, chopped
- 1/4 cup extra-virgin olive oil
- 2 tbsp red wine vinegar
- 2 tbsp lemon juice
- 1/4 tsp cayenne pepper
- Sea salt and freshly ground black pepper, to season
- 1 avocado, peeled, pitted and sliced
- 1 tbsp sesame seeds, toasted

Directions:
- Place the water and quinoa in a saucepan and bring it to a rolling boil. Immediately turn the heat to a simmer.
- Let it simmer for about 13 minutes until the quinoa has absorbed all of the water; fluff the quinoa with a fork and let it cool completely. Then, transfer the quinoa to a salad bowl.
- Add the onion, tomato, roasted peppers, parsley and basil to the salad bowl. In another small bowl, whisk the olive oil, vinegar, lemon juice, cayenne pepper, salt and black pepper.
- Dress your salad and toss to combine well. Top with avocado slices and garnish with toasted sesame seeds.
- Enjoy

64) VEGETARIAN TABBOULEH SALAD WITH TOFU

Preparation Time: 20 minutes + chilling time		Servings: 4
Ingredients: - 1 cup bulgur wheat - 2 San Marzano tomatoes, sliced - 1 Persian cucumber, thinly sliced - 2 tbsp basil, chopped - 2 tbsp parsley, chopped - 4 scallions, chopped - 2 cups arugula	- 2 cups baby spinach, torn into pieces - 4 tbsp tahini - 4 tbsp lemon juice - 1 tbsp soy sauce - 1 tsp fresh garlic, pressed - Sea salt and ground black pepper, to taste - 12 ounces smoked tofu, cubed	**Directions:** - In a saucepan, bring 2 cups of water and the bulgur to a boil. Immediately turn the heat to a simmer and let it cook for about 20 minutes or until the bulgur is tender and the water is almost absorbed. Fluff with a fork and spread on a large tray to let cool. - Place the bulgur in a salad bowl followed by the tomatoes, cucumber, basil, parsley, scallions, arugula and spinach. - In a small mixing dish, whisk the tahini, lemon juice, soy sauce, garlic, salt and black pepper. Dress the salad and toss to combine. - Top your salad with the smoked tofu and serve at room temperature. Enjoy

65) SPECIAL GREEN PASTA SALAD

Preparation Time: 10 minutes + chilling time		Servings: 4
Ingredients: - 12 ounces rotini pasta - 1 small onion, thinly sliced - 1 cup cherry tomatoes, halved - 1 bell pepper, chopped - 1 jalapeno pepper, chopped - 1 tbsp capers, drained - 2 cups Iceberg lettuce, torn into pieces - 2 tbsp fresh parsley, chopped	- 2 tbsp fresh cilantro, chopped - 2 tbsp fresh basil, chopped - 1/4 cup olive oil - 2 tbsp apple cider vinegar - 1 tsp garlic, pressed - Kosher salt and ground black pepper, to taste - 2 tbsp nutritional yeast - 2 tbsp pine nuts, toasted and chopped	**Directions:** - Cook the pasta according to the package directions. Drain and rinse the pasta. Let it cool completely and then, transfer it to a salad bowl. - Then, add in the onion, tomatoes, peppers, capers, lettuce, parsley, cilantro and basil to the salad bowl. - Whisk the olive oil, vinegar, garlic, salt, black pepper and nutritional yeast. Dress your salad and top with toasted pine nuts. Enjoy

Chapter 3. DINNER

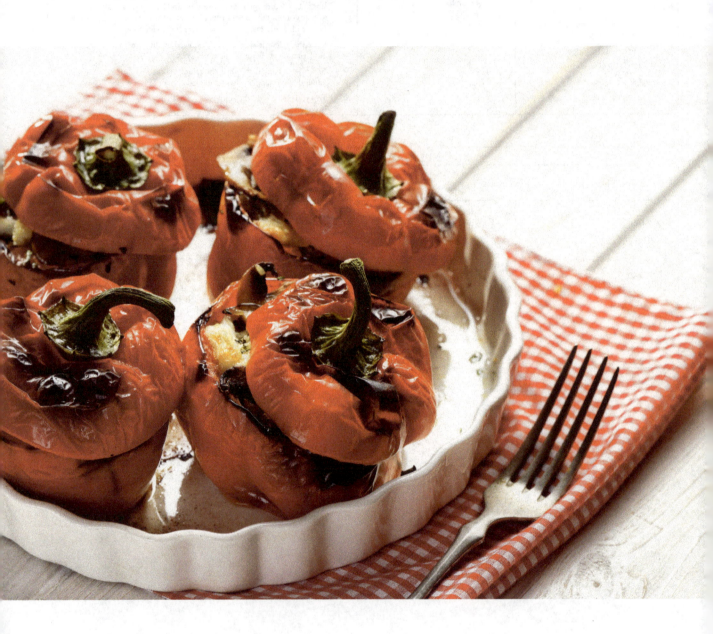

66) AUTHENTIC UKRAINIAN BORSCHT

Preparation Time: 40 minutes **Servings:** 4

Ingredients:
- 2 tbsp sesame oil
- 1 red onion, chopped
- 2 carrots, trimmed and sliced
- 2 large beets, peeled and sliced
- 2 large potatoes, peeled and diced
- 4 cups vegetable stock
- 2 garlic cloves, minced
- 1/2 tsp caraway seeds
- 1/2 tsp celery seeds
- 1/2 tsp fennel seeds
- 1 pound red cabbage, shredded
- 1/2 tsp mixed peppercorns, freshly cracked
- Kosher salt, to taste
- 2 bay leaves
- 2 tbsp wine vinegar

Directions:
- In a Dutch oven, heat the sesame oil over a moderate flame. Once hot, sauté the onions until tender and translucent, about 6 minutes.
- Add in the carrots, beets and potatoes and continue to sauté an additional 10 minutes, adding the vegetable stock periodically.
- Next, stir in the garlic, caraway seeds, celery seeds, fennel seeds and continue sautéing for another 30 seconds.
- Add in the cabbage, mixed peppercorns, salt and bay leaves. Add in the remaining stock and bring to boil.
- Immediately turn the heat to a simmer and continue to cook for 20 to 23 minutes longer until the vegetables have softened.
- Ladle into individual bowls and drizzle wine vinegar over it. Serve and enjoy

67) MOROCCAN LENTIL BELUGA SALAD

Preparation Time: 20 minutes + chilling time **Servings:** 4

Ingredients:
- 1 cup Beluga lentils, rinsed
- 1 Persian cucumber, sliced
- 1 large-sized tomatoes, sliced
- 1 red onion, chopped
- 1 bell pepper, sliced
- 1/4 cup fresh basil, chopped
- 1/4 cup fresh Italian parsley, chopped
- 2 ounces green olives, pitted and sliced
- 1/4 cup olive oil
- 4 tbsp lemon juice
- 1 tsp deli mustard
- 1/2 tsp garlic, minced
- 1/2 tsp red pepper flakes, crushed
- Sea salt and ground black pepper, to taste

Directions:
- In a large-sized saucepan, bring 3 cups of the water and 1 cup of the lentils to a boil.
- Immediately turn the heat to a simmer and continue to cook your lentils for a further 15 to 17 minutes or until they've softened but not mushy. Drain and let it cool completely.
- Transfer the lentils to a salad bowl; add in the cucumber, tomatoes, onion, pepper, basil, parsley and olives.
- In a small mixing dish, whisk the olive oil, lemon juice, mustard, garlic, red pepper, salt and black pepper.
- Dress the salad, toss to combine and serve well-chilled. Enjoy

68) INDIAN-STYLE NAAN SALAD

Preparation Time: 10 minutes **Servings:** 3

Ingredients:
- 3 tbsp sesame oil
- 1 tsp ginger, peeled and minced
- 1/2 tsp cumin seeds
- 1/2 tsp mustard seeds
- 1/2 tsp mixed peppercorns
- 1 tbsp curry leaves
- 3 naan breads, broken into bite-sized pieces
- 1 shallot, chopped
- 2 tomatoes, chopped
- Himalayan salt, to taste
- 1 tbsp soy sauce

Directions:
- Heat 2 tbsp of the sesame oil in a non-stick skillet over a moderately high heat.
- Sauté the ginger, cumin seeds, mustard seeds, mixed peppercorns and curry leaves for 1 minute or so, until fragrant.
- Stir in the naan breads and continue to cook, stirring periodically, until golden-brown and well coated with the spices.
- Place the shallot and tomatoes in a salad bowl; toss them with the salt, soy sauce and the remaining 1 tbsp of the sesame oil.
- Place the toasted naan on the top of your salad and serve at room temperature. Enjoy

69) ITALIAN BROCCOLI GINGER SOUP

Preparation Time: 50 minutes   **Servings:** 4

Ingredients:
- 1 onion, chopped
- 1 tbsp minced peeled fresh ginger
- 2 tsp olive oil
- 2 carrots, chopped
- 1 head broccoli, chopped into florets
- 1 cup coconut milk
- 3 cups vegetable broth
- ½ tsp turmeric
- Salt and black pepper to taste

Directions:
- In a pot over medium heat, place the onion, ginger, and olive oil, cook for 4 minutes. Add in carrots, broccoli, broth, turmeric, pepper, and salt. Bring to a boil and cook for 15 minutes. Transfer the soup to a food processor and blend until smooth. Stir in coconut milk and serve warm

70) ASIAN NOODLE RICE SOUP WITH BEANS

Preparation Time: 10 minutes   **Servings:** 6

Ingredients:
- 2 carrots, chopped
- 2 celery stalks, chopped
- 6 cups vegetable broth
- 8 oz brown rice noodles
- 1 (15-oz) can pinto beans
- 1 tsp dried herbs

Directions:
- Place a pot over medium heat and add in the carrots, celery, and vegetable broth. Bring to a boil. Add in noodles, beans, dried herbs, salt, and pepper. Reduce the heat and simmer for 5 minutes. Serve

71) SPECIAL VEGETABLE AND RICE SOUP

Preparation Time: 40 minutes   **Servings:** 6

Ingredients:
- 3 tbsp olive oil
- 2 carrots, chopped
- 1 onion, chopped
- 1 celery stalk, chopped
- 2 garlic cloves, minced
- 2 cups chopped cabbage
- ½ red bell pepper, chopped
- 4 potatoes, unpeeled and quartered
- 6 cups vegetable broth
- ½ cup brown rice, rinsed
- ½ cup frozen green peas
- 2 tbsp chopped parsley

Directions:
- Heat the oil in a pot over medium heat. Place carrots, onion, celery, and garlic. Cook for 5 minutes. Add in cabbage, bell pepper, potatoes, and broth. Bring to a boil, then lower the heat and add the brown rice, salt, and pepper. Simmer uncovered for 25 minutes until vegetables are tender. Stir in peas and cook for 5 minutes. Top with parsley and serve warm

72) EASY DAIKON AND SWEET POTATO SOUP

Preparation Time: 40 minutes   **Servings:** 6

Ingredients:
- 6 cups water
- 2 tsp olive oil
- 1 chopped onion
- 3 garlic cloves, minced
- 1 tbsp thyme
- 2 tsp paprika
- 2 cups peeled and chopped daikon
- 2 cups chopped sweet potatoes
- 2 cups peeled and chopped parsnips
- ½ tsp sea salt
- 1 cup fresh mint, chopped
- ½ avocado
- 2 tbsp balsamic vinegar
- 2 tbsp pumpkin seeds

Directions:
- Heat the oil in a pot and place onion and garlic. Sauté for 3 minutes. Add in thyme, paprika, daikon, sweet potato, parsnips, water, and salt. Bring to a boil and cook for 30 minutes. Remove the soup to a food processor and add in balsamic vinegar; purée until smooth. Top with mint and pumpkin seeds to serve

73) TASTY CHICKPEA AND VEGETABLE SOUP

Preparation Time: 35 minutes

Servings: 5

Ingredients:

- 2 tbsp olive oil
- 1 onion, chopped
- 1 carrot, chopped
- 1 celery stalk, chopped
- 1 eggplant, chopped
- 1 (28-oz) can diced tomatoes
- 2 tbsp tomato paste
- 1 (15.5-oz) can chickpeas, drained
- 2 tsp smoked paprika
- 1 tsp ground cumin
- 1 tsp za'atar spice
- ¼ tsp ground cayenne pepper
- 6 cups vegetable broth
- 4 oz whole-wheat vermicelli
- 2 tbsp minced cilantro

Directions:

- Heat the oil in a pot over medium heat. Place onion, carrot, and celery and cook for 5 minutes. Add in eggplant, tomatoes, tomato paste, chickpeas, paprika, cumin, za´atar spice, and cayenne pepper. Stir in broth and salt. Bring to a boil, then lower the heat and simmer for 15 minutes. Add in vermicelli and cook for another 5 minutes. Serve topped with cilantro

74) ITALIAN-STYLE BEAN SOUP

Preparation Time: 1 hour 25 minutes

Servings: 6

Ingredients:

- 3 tbsp olive oil
- 2 celery stalks, chopped
- 2 carrots, chopped
- 3 shallots, chopped
- 3 garlic cloves, minced
- ½ cup brown rice
- 6 cups vegetable broth
- 1 (14.5-oz) can diced tomatoes
- 2 bay leaves
- Salt and black pepper to taste
- 2 (15.5-oz) cans white beans
- ¼ cup chopped basil

Directions:

- Heat oil in a pot over medium heat. Place celery, carrots, shallots, and garlic and cook for 5 minutes. Add in brown rice, broth, tomatoes, bay leaves, salt, and pepper. Bring to a boil, then lower the heat and simmer uncovered for 20 minutes. Stir in beans and basil and cook for 5 minutes. Discard bay leaves and spoon into bowls. Sprinkle with basil and serve

75) LOVELY BRUSSELS SPROUTS AND TOFU SOUP

Preparation Time: 40 minutes

Servings: 4

Ingredients:

- 7 oz firm tofu, cubed
- 2 tsp olive oil
- 1 cup sliced mushrooms
- 1 cup shredded Brussels sprouts
- 1 garlic clove, minced
- ½-inch piece fresh ginger, minced
- Salt to taste
- 2 tbsp apple cider vinegar
- 2 tbsp soy sauce
- 1 tsp pure date sugar
- ¼ tsp red pepper flakes
- 1 scallion, chopped

Directions:

- Heat the oil in a skillet over medium heat. Place mushrooms, Brussels sprouts, garlic, ginger, and salt. Sauté for 7-8 minutes until the veggies are soft. Pour in 4 cups of water, vinegar, soy sauce, sugar, pepper flakes, and tofu. Bring to a boil, then lower the heat and simmer for 5-10 minutes. Top with scallions and serve

76) CREAMY WHITE BEAN ROSEMARY SOUP

Preparation Time: 30 minutes | **Servings:** 4

Ingredients:
- 2 tsp olive oil
- 1 carrot, chopped
- 1 onion, chopped
- 2 garlic cloves, minced
- 1 tbsp rosemary, chopped
- 2 tbsp apple cider vinegar
- 1 cup dried white beans
- ¼ tsp salt
- 2 tbsp nutritional yeast

Directions:
- Heat the oil in a pot over medium heat. Place carrots, onion, and garlic and cook for 5 minutes.
- Pour in vinegar to deglaze the pot. Stir in 5 cups water and beans and bring to a boil. Lower the heat and simmer for 45 minutes until the beans are soft. Add in salt and nutritional yeast and stir. Serve topped with chopped rosemary

77) DELICIOUS MUSHROOM AND TOFU SOUP

Preparation Time: 20 minutes | **Servings:** 4

Ingredients:
- 4 cups water
- 2 tbsp soy sauce
- 4 white mushrooms, sliced
- ¼ cup chopped green onions
- 3 tbsp tahini
- 6 oz extra-firm tofu, diced

Directions:
- Pour the water and soy sauce into a pot and bring to a boil. Add in mushrooms and green onions. Lower the heat and simmer for 10 minutes. In a bowl, combine ½ cup of hot soup with tahini. Pour the mixture into the pot and simmer 2 minutes more, but not boil. Stir in tofu. Serve warm

78) TROPICAL COCONUT CREAM BUTTERNUT SQUASH SOUP

Preparation Time: 30 minutes | **Servings:** 5

Ingredients:
- 1 (2-lb) butternut squash, cubed
- 1 red bell pepper, chopped
- 1 large onion, chopped
- 3 garlic cloves, minced
- 4 cups vegetable broth
- 1 cup coconut cream

Directions:
- Place the squash, bell pepper, onion, garlic, and broth in a pot. Bring to a boil. Lower the heat and simmer for 20 minutes. Stir in coconut cream, salt and pepper. Transfer to a food processor purée the soup until smooth. Serve warm

79) ITALIAN MUSHROOM COCONUT SOUP

Preparation Time: 20 minutes | **Servings:** 2

Ingredients:
- 2 tsp olive oil
- 1 onion, chopped
- 2 garlic cloves, minced
- 2 cups chopped mushrooms
- Salt and black pepper to taste
- 2 tbsp whole-wheat flour
- 1 tsp dried rosemary
- 4 cups vegetable broth
- 1 cup coconut cream

Directions:
- In a pot over medium heat, warm the oil. Place the onion, garlic, mushrooms, and salt and cook for 5 minutes. Stir in the flour and cook for another 1-2 minutes. Add in rosemary, vegetable broth, coconut cream, and pepper. Lower the heat and simmer for 10 minutes. Serve

80) GREEK TOMATO CREAM SOUP

Preparation Time: 15 minutes

Servings: 5

Ingredients:
- 1 (28-oz) can tomatoes
- 2 tbsp olive oil
- 1 tsp smoked paprika
- 2 cups vegetable broth
- 2 tsp dried herbs
- 1 red onion, chopped
- 1 cup unsweetened non-dairy milk
- Salt and black pepper to taste

Directions:
- Place the tomatoes, olive oil, paprika, broth, dried herbs, onion, milk, salt, and pepper in a pot. Bring to a boil and cook for 10 minutes. Transfer to a food processor and blend the soup until smooth

81) SPECIAL ROASTED PEPPER SALAD IN GREEK-STYLE

Preparation Time: 10 minutes

Servings: 2

Ingredients:
- 2 red bell peppers
- 2 yellow bell peppers
- 2 garlic cloves, pressed
- 4 tsp extra-virgin olive oil
- 1 tbsp capers, rinsed and drained
- 2 tbsp red wine vinegar
- Seas salt and ground pepper, to taste
- 1 tsp fresh dill weed, chopped
- 1 tsp fresh oregano, chopped
- 1/4 cup Kalamata olives, pitted and sliced

Directions:
- Broil the peppers on a parchment-lined baking sheet for about 10 minutes, rotating the pan halfway through the cooking time, until they are charred on all sides.
- Then, cover the peppers with a plastic wrap to steam. Discard the skin, seeds and cores.
- Slice the peppers into strips and place them in a salad bowl. Add in the remaining ingredients and toss to combine well.
- Place in your refrigerator until ready to serve. Enjoy

82) SWEET POTATO AND KIDNEY BEAN SOUP

Preparation Time: 30 minutes

Servings: 4

Ingredients:
- 2 tbsp olive oil
- 1 onion, chopped
- 1 pound potatoes, peeled and diced
- 1 medium celery stalks, chopped
- 2 garlic cloves, minced
- 1 tsp paprika
- 4 cups water
- 2 tbsp vegan bouillon powder
- 16 ounces canned kidney beans, drained
- 2 cups baby spinach
- Sea salt and ground black pepper, to taste

Directions:
- In a heavy-bottomed pot, heat the olive over medium-high heat. Now, sauté the onion, potatoes and celery for approximately 5 minutes or until the onion is translucent and tender.
- Add in the garlic and continue to sauté for 1 minute or until aromatic.
- Then, add in the paprika, water and vegan bouillon powder and bring to a boil. Immediately reduce the heat to a simmer and let it cook for 15 minutes.
- Fold in the navy beans and spinach; continue to simmer for about 5 minutes until everything is thoroughly heated. Season with salt and black pepper to taste.
- Ladle into individual bowls and serve hot. Enjoy

83) WINTER QUINOA SALAD WITH PICKLES

Preparation Time: 20 minutes + chilling time		Servings: 4

Ingredients:
- 1 cup quinoa
- 4 garlic cloves, minced
- 2 pickled cucumber, chopped
- 10 ounces canned red peppers, chopped
- 1/2 cup green olives, pitted and sliced
- 2 cups green cabbages, shredded
- 2 cups Iceberg lettuce, torn into pieces
- 4 pickled chilies, chopped
- 4 tbsp olive oil
- 1 tbsp lemon juice
- 1 tsp lemon zest
- 1/2 tsp dried marjoram
- Sea salt and ground black pepper, to taste
- 1/4 cup fresh chives, coarsely chopped

Directions:
- Place two cups of water and the quinoa in a pot and bring it to a boil. Immediately turn the heat to a simmer.
- Let it simmer for about 13 minutes until the quinoa has absorbed all of the water; fluff the quinoa with a fork and let it cool completely. Then, transfer the quinoa to a salad bowl.
- Add the garlic, pickled cucumber, peppers, olives, cabbage, lettuce and pickled chilies to the salad bowl and toss to combine.
- In a small mixing bowl, make the dressing by whisking the remaining ingredients. Dress the salad, toss to combine well and serve immediately. Enjoy

84) SUPER WILD ROASTED MUSHROOM SOUP

Preparation Time: 55 minutes		Servings: 3

Ingredients:
- 3 tbsp sesame oil
- 1 pound mixed wild mushrooms, sliced
- 1 white onion, chopped
- 3 cloves garlic, minced and divided
- 2 sprigs thyme, chopped
- 2 sprigs rosemary, chopped
- 1/4 cup flaxseed meal
- 1/4 cup dry white wine
- 3 cups vegetable broth
- 1/2 tsp red chili flakes
- Garlic salt and freshly ground black pepper, to seasoned

Directions:
- Start by preheating your oven to 395 degrees F.
- Place the mushrooms in a single layer onto a parchment-lined baking pan. Drizzle the mushrooms with 1 tbsp of the sesame oil.
- Roast the mushrooms in the preheated oven for about 25 minutes, or until tender.
- Heat the remaining 2 tbsp of the sesame oil in a stockpot over medium heat. Then, sauté the onion for about 3 minutes or until tender and translucent.
- Then, add in the garlic, thyme and rosemary and continue to sauté for 1 minute or so until aromatic. Sprinkle flaxseed meal over everything.
- Add in the remaining ingredients and continue to simmer for 10 to 15 minutes longer or until everything is cooked through.
- Stir in the roasted mushrooms and continue simmering for a further 12 minutes. Ladle into soup bowls and serve hot. Enjoy

85) SPECIAL GREEN BEAN SOUP IN MEDITERRANEAN-STYLE

Preparation Time: 25 minutes		Servings: 5

Ingredients:
- 2 tbsp olive oil
- 1 onion, chopped
- 1 celery with leaves, chopped
- 1 carrot, chopped
- 2 garlic cloves, minced
- 1 zucchini, chopped
- 5 cups vegetable broth
- 1 ¼ pounds green beans, trimmed and cut into bite-sized chunks
- 2 medium-sized tomatoes, pureed
- Sea salt and freshly ground black pepper, to taste
- 1/2 tsp cayenne pepper
- 1 tsp oregano
- 1/2 tsp dried dill
- 1/2 cup Kalamata olives, pitted and sliced

Directions:
- In a heavy-bottomed pot, heat the olive over medium-high heat. Now, sauté the onion, celery and carrot for about 4 minutes or until the vegetables are just tender.
- Add in the garlic and zucchini and continue to sauté for 1 minute or until aromatic.
- Then, stir in the vegetable broth, green beans, tomatoes, salt, black pepper, cayenne pepper, oregano and dried dill; bring to a boil. Immediately reduce the heat to a simmer and let it cook for about 15 minutes.
- Ladle into individual bowls and serve with sliced olives. Enjoy

86) LOVELY CREAMY CARROT SOUP

Preparation Time: 30 minutes

Servings: 4

Ingredients:
- 2 tbsp sesame oil
- 1 onion, chopped
- 1 ½ pounds carrots, trimmed and chopped
- 1 parsnip, chopped
- 2 garlic cloves, minced
- 1/2 tsp curry powder
- Sea salt and cayenne pepper, to taste
- 4 cups vegetable broth
- 1 cup full-fat coconut milk

Directions:
- In a heavy-bottomed pot, heat the sesame oil over medium-high heat. Now, sauté the onion, carrots and parsnip for about 5 minutes, stirring periodically.
- Add in the garlic and continue sautéing for 1 minute or until fragrant.
- Then, stir in the curry powder, salt, cayenne pepper and vegetable broth; bring to a rapid boil. Immediately reduce the heat to a simmer and let it cook for 18 to 20 minutes.
- Puree the soup using an immersion blender until creamy and uniform.
- Return the pureed mixture to the pot. Fold in the coconut milk and continue to simmer until heated through or about 5 minutes longer.
- Ladle into four bowls and serve hot. Enjoy

87) SPECIAL ITALIAN NONNO'S PIZZA SALAD

Preparation Time: 15 minutes + chilling time

Servings: 4

Ingredients:
- 1 pound macaroni
- 1 cup marinated mushrooms, sliced
- 1 cup grape tomatoes, halved
- 4 tbsp scallions, chopped
- 1 tsp garlic, minced
- 1 Italian pepper, sliced
- 1/4 cup extra-virgin olive oil
- 1/4 cup balsamic vinegar
- 1 tsp dried oregano
- 1 tsp dried basil
- 1/2 tsp dried rosemary
- Sea salt and cayenne pepper, to taste
- 1/2 cup black olives, sliced

Directions:
- Cook the pasta according to the package directions. Drain and rinse the pasta. Let it cool completely and then, transfer it to a salad bowl.
- Then, add in the remaining ingredients and toss until the macaroni are well coated.
- Taste and adjust the seasonings; place the pizza salad in your refrigerator until ready to use. Enjoy

88) SPECIAL CREAM OF GOLDEN VEGGIE SOUP

Preparation Time: 45 minutes

Servings: 4

Ingredients:
- 2 tbsp avocado oil
- 1 yellow onion, chopped
- 2 Yukon Gold potatoes, peeled and diced
- 2 pounds butternut squash, peeled, seeded and diced
- 1 parsnip, trimmed and sliced
- 1 tsp ginger-garlic paste
- 1 tsp turmeric powder
- 1 tsp fennel seeds
- 1/2 tsp chili powder
- 1/2 tsp pumpkin pie spice
- Kosher salt and ground black pepper, to taste
- 3 cups vegetable stock
- 1 cup full-fat coconut milk
- 2 tbsp pepitas

Directions:
- In a heavy-bottomed pot, heat the oil over medium-high heat. Now, sauté the onion, potatoes, butternut squash and parsnip for about 10 minutes, stirring periodically to ensure even cooking.
- Add in the ginger-garlic paste and continue sautéing for 1 minute or until aromatic.
- Then, stir in the turmeric powder, fennel seeds, chili powder, pumpkin pie spice, salt, black pepper and vegetable stock; bring to a boil. Immediately reduce the heat to a simmer and let it cook for about 25 minutes.
- Puree the soup using an immersion blender until creamy and uniform.
- Return the pureed mixture to the pot. Fold in the coconut milk and continue to simmer until heated through or about 5 minutes longer.
- Ladle into individual bowls and serve garnished with pepitas. Enjoy

89) EASY ROASTED CAULIFLOWER SOUP

Preparation Time: 1 hour

Servings: 4

Ingredients:
- 1 ½ pounds cauliflower florets
- 4 tbsp olive oil
- 1 onion, chopped
- 2 cloves garlic, minced
- 1/2 tsp ginger, peeled and minced
- 1 tsp fresh rosemary, chopped
- 2 tbsp fresh basil, chopped
- 2 tbsp fresh parsley, chopped
- 4 cups vegetable stock
- Sea salt and ground black pepper, to taste
- 1/2 tsp ground sumac
- 1/4 cup tahini
- 1 lemon, freshly squeezed

Directions:
- Begin by preheating the oven to 425 degrees F. Toss the cauliflower with 2 tbsp of the olive oil and arrange them on a parchment-lined roasting pan.
- Then, roast the cauliflower florets for about 30 minutes stirring, them once or twice to promote even cooking.
- Meanwhile, in a heavy-bottomed pot, heat the remaining 2 tbsp of the olive oil over medium-high heat. Now, sauté the onion for about 4 minutes until tender and translucent.
- Add in the garlic, ginger, rosemary, basil and parsley and continue sautéing for 1 minute or until fragrant.
- Then, stir in the vegetable stock, salt, black pepper and sumac and bring it to a boil. Immediately reduce the heat to a simmer and let it cook for about 20 to 22 minutes.
- Puree the soup using an immersion blender until creamy and uniform.
- Return the pureed mixture to the pot. Fold in the tahini and continue to simmer for about 5 minutes or until everything is thoroughly cooked.
- Ladle into individual bowls, garnish with lemon juice and serve hot. Enjoy

90) AUTHENTIC VEGAN COLESLAW

Preparation Time: 10 minutes

Servings: 4

Ingredients:
- 1 pound red cabbage, shredded
- 2 carrots, trimmed and grated
- 4 tbsp onion, chopped
- 1 garlic clove, minced
- 1/2 cup fresh Italian parsley, roughly chopped
- 1 cup vegan mayo
- 1 tsp brown mustard
- 1 tsp lemon zest
- 2 tbsp apple cider vinegar
- Sea salt and ground black pepper, to taste
- 2 tbsp sunflower seeds

Directions:
- Toss the cabbage, carrots, onion, garlic and parsley in a salad bowl.
- In a mixing bowl, whisk the mayo, mustard, lemon zest, apple cider vinegar, salt and black pepper.
- Dress your salad and serve garnished with the sunflower seeds

91) SUPER HOT COLLARD SALAD

Preparation Time: 10 minutes

Servings: 2

Ingredients:
- ¾ cup coconut whipping cream
- 2 tbsp tofu mayonnaise
- A pinch of mustard powder
- 2 tbsp coconut oil
- 1 garlic clove, minced
- Salt and black pepper to taste
- 2 oz plant butter
- 1 cup collards, rinsed
- 4 oz tofu cheese

Directions:
- In a small bowl, whisk the coconut whipping cream, tofu mayonnaise, mustard powder, coconut oil, garlic, salt, and black pepper until well mixed; set aside. Melt the plant butter in a large skillet over medium heat and sauté the collards until wilted and brownish. Season with salt and black pepper to taste. Transfer the collards to a salad bowl and pour the creamy dressing over. Mix the salad well and crumble the tofu cheese over. Serve

92) SUPER ROASTED MUSHROOMS AND GREEN BEANS SALAD

Preparation Time: 25 minutes

Servings: 4

Ingredients:
- 1 lb. cremini mushrooms, sliced
- ½ cup green beans
- 3 tbsp melted plant butter
- Salt and black pepper to taste
- Juice of 1 lemon
- 4 tbsp toasted hazelnuts

Directions:
- Preheat oven to 450 F.
- Arrange the mushrooms and green beans in a baking dish, drizzle the plant butter over, and sprinkle with salt and black pepper. Use your hands to rub the vegetables with the seasoning and roast in the oven for 20 minutes or until they are soft. Transfer the vegetables into a salad bowl, drizzle with the lemon juice, and toss the salad with the hazelnuts. Serve the salad immediately

93) MEXICAN BEAN AND COUSCOUS SALAD

Preparation Time: 15 minutes

Servings: 4

Ingredients:
- ¼ cup olive oil
- 1 medium shallot, minced
- ½ tsp ground coriander
- ½ tsp turmeric
- ¼ tsp ground cayenne
- 1 cup couscous
- 2 cups vegetable broth
- 1 yellow bell pepper, chopped
- 1 carrot, shredded
- ½ cup chopped dried apricots
- ¼ cup golden raisins
- ¼ cup chopped roasted cashews
- 1 (15.5-oz) can white beans
- 2 tbsp minced fresh cilantro leaves
- 2 tbsp fresh lemon juice

Directions:
- Heat 1 tbsp of oil in a pot over medium heat. Place in shallot, coriander, turmeric, cayenne pepper, and couscous. Cook for 2 minutes, stirring often. Add in broth and salt. Bring to a boil. Turn the heat off and let sit covered for 5 minutes. Remove to a bowl and stir in bell pepper, carrot, apricots, raisins, cashews, beans, and cilantro. Set aside. In another bowl, whisk the remaining oil with lemon juice until blended. Pour over the salad and toss to combine. Serve immediately

94) VEGETARIAN SEITAN AND SPINACH SALAD A LA PUTTANESCA

Preparation Time: 11 minutes

Servings: 4

Ingredients:
- 4 tbsp olive oil
- 8 oz seitan, cut into strips
- 2 garlic cloves, minced
- ½ cup Kalamata olives, halved
- ½ cup green olives, halved
- 2 tbsp capers
- 3 cups baby spinach, cut into strips
- 1 ½ cups cherry tomatoes, halved
- 2 tbsp balsamic vinegar
- 2 tbsp torn fresh basil leaves
- 2 tbsp minced fresh parsley
- 1 cup pomegranate seeds

Directions:
- Heat half of the olive oil in a skillet over medium heat. Place the seitan and brown for 5 minutes on all sides. Add in garlic and cook for 30 seconds. Remove to a bowl and let cool. Stir in olives, capers, spinach, and tomatoes. Set aside.
- In another bowl, whisk the remaining oil, vinegar, salt, and pepper until well mixed. Pour this dressing over the seitan salad and toss to coat. Top with basil, parsley, and pomegranate seeds. Serve

95) POMODORO AND AVOCADO LETTUCE SALAD

Preparation Time: 15 minutes

Servings: 4

Ingredients:
- 1 garlic clove, chopped
- 1 red onion, sliced
- ½ tsp dried basil
- Salt and black pepper to taste
- ¼ tsp pure date sugar
- 3 tbsp white wine vinegar
- 1/3 cup olive oil
- 1 head Iceberg lettuce, shredded
- 12 ripe grape tomatoes, halved
- ½ cup frozen peas, thawed
- 8 black olives, pitted
- 1 avocado, sliced

Directions:
- In a food processor, place the garlic, onion, oil, basil, salt, pepper, sugar, and vinegar. Blend until smooth. Set aside. Place the lettuce, tomatoes, peas, and olives on a nice serving plate. Top with avocado slices and drizzle the previously prepared dressing all over. Serve

96) SPECIAL FRIED BROCCOLI SALAD WITH TEMPEH AND CRANBERRIES

Preparation Time: 15 minutes

Servings: 4

Ingredients:
- 3 oz plant butter
- ¾ lb tempeh slices, cubed
- 1 lb broccoli florets
- Salt and black pepper to taste
- 2 oz almonds
- ½ cup frozen cranberries

Directions:
- In a skillet, melt the plant butter over medium heat until no longer foaming, and fry the tempeh cubes until brown on all sides. Add the broccoli and stir-fry for 6 minutes. Season with salt and pepper. Turn the heat off. Stir in the almonds and cranberries to warm through. Share salad into bowls and serve

97) HEALTHY BALSAMIC LENTIL SALAD

Preparation Time: 40 minutes

Servings: 4

Ingredients:
- 2 tsp olive oil
- 1 red onion, diced
- 1 garlic clove, minced
- 1 carrot, diced
- 1 cup lentils
- 1 tbsp dried basil
- 1 tbsp dried oregano
- 1 tbsp balsamic vinegar
- 2 cups water
- Sea salt to taste
- 2 cups chopped Swiss chard
- 2 cups torn curly endive

Directions:
- In a bowl, mix the balsamic vinegar, olive oil, and salt. Set aside. Warm 1 tsp of oil in a pot over medium heat. Place the onion and carrot and cook for 5 minutes. Mix in lentils, basil, oregano, balsamic vinegar, and water and bring to a boil. Lower the heat and simmer for 20 minutes.
- Mix in two-thirds of the dressing. Add in the Swiss chard and cook for 5 minutes on low. Let cool. Coat the endive with the remaining dressing. Transfer to a plate and top with lentil mixture to serve

98) SUPER HOT GREEN BEAN AND POTATO SALAD

Preparation Time: 25 minutes

Servings: 4

Ingredients:
- Salt and black pepper to taste
- 1 cup green beans, chopped
- 4 potatoes, quartered
- 2 carrots, sliced
- 1 tbsp extra-virgin olive oil
- 1 tbsp lime juice
- 2 tsp dried dill
- 1 cup cashew cream

Directions:
- Pour salted water in a pot over medium heat. Add in potatoes, bring to a boil and cook for 8 minutes. Put in carrots and green beans and cook for 8 minutes. Drain and put in a bowl. Mix in olive oil, lime juice, dill, cashew cream, salt, and pepper. Toss to coat. Allow cooling before serving

99) EASY MILLET SALAD WITH OLIVES AND CHERRIES

Preparation Time: 40 minutes **Servings:** 4

Ingredients:
- 1 cup millet
- 1 (15.5-oz) can navy beans
- 1 celery stalk, finely chopped
- 1 carrot, shredded
- 3 green onions, minced
- ½ cup chopped kalamata olives
- ½ cup dried cherries
- ½ cup toasted pecans, chopped
- ½ cup minced fresh parsley
- 1 garlic clove, pressed
- 3 tbsp sherry vinegar
- ¼ cup grapeseed oil

Directions:
- Cook the millet in salted water for 30 minutes. Remove to a bowl. Mix in beans, celery, carrot, green onions, olives, cherries, pecans, and parsley. Set aside. In another bowl, whisk the garlic, vinegar, salt, and pepper until well mixed. Pour over the millet mixture and toss to coat. Serve immediately

100) DELICIOUS DAIKON SALAD WITH CARAMELIZED ONION

Preparation Time: 50 minutes **Servings:** 4

Ingredients:
- 1 lb daikon, peeled
- 2 cups sliced sweet onions
- 2 tsp olive oil
- Salt to taste
- 1 tbsp rice vinegar

Directions:
- Place the daikon in a pot with salted water and cook 25 minutes, until tender. Drain and let cool. In a skillet over low heat, warm olive oil and add the onion. Sauté for 10-15 minutes until caramelized. Sprinkle with salt. Remove to a bowl. Chop the daikon into wedges and add to the onion bowl. Stir in the vinegar. Serve

101) BLACK CABBAGE AND BEET SALAD

Cooking Time: 50 Minutes **Servings:** 6

- 1 bunch of kale, washed and dried, ribs removed, chopped
- 6 pieces washed beets, peeled and dried and cut into ½ inches
- ½ tsp dried rosemary
- ½ tsp garlic powder
- salt
- pepper
- olive oil
- ¼ medium red onion, thinly sliced
- 1-2 tbsp slivered almonds, toasted
- ¼ cup olive oil
- Juice of 1½ lemon
- ¼ cup honey
- ¼ tsp garlic powder
- 1 tsp dried rosemary
- salt
- pepper

- Preheat oven to 400 degrees F.
- Take a bowl and toss the kale with some salt, pepper, and olive oil.
- Lightly oil a baking sheet and add the kale.
- Roast in the oven for 5 minutes, and then remove and place to the side.
- Place beets in a bowl and sprinkle with a bit of rosemary, garlic powder, pepper, and salt; ensure beets are coated well.
- Spread the beets on the oiled baking sheet, place on the middle rack of your oven, and roast for 45 minutes, turning twice.
- Make the lemon vinaigrette by whisking all of the listed Ingredients: in a bowl.
- Once the beets are ready, remove from the oven and allow it to cool.
- Take a medium-sized salad bowl and add kale, onions, and beets.
- Dress with lemon honey vinaigrette and toss well.
- Garnish with toasted almonds.
- Enjoy!

102) POMODORO LETTUCE SALAD

Cooking Time: 15 Minutes **Servings:** 6

Ingredients	Ingredients	Directions
- 1 heart of Romaine lettuce, chopped - 3 Roma tomatoes, diced - 1 English cucumber, diced - 1 small red onion, finely chopped - ½ cup curly parsley, finely chopped	- 2 tbsp virgin olive oil - lemon juice, ½ large lemon - 1 tsp garlic powder - salt - pepper	- Add all Ingredients: to a large bowl. - Toss well and transfer them to containers. - Enjoy!

103) Avocado Arugula Salad

Cooking Time: 15 Minutes **Servings:** 4

Ingredients	Ingredients	Directions
- 4 cups packed baby arugula - 4 green onions, tops trimmed, chopped - 1½ cups shelled fava beans - 3 Persian cucumbers, chopped - 2 cups grape tomatoes, halved - 1 jalapeno pepper, sliced - 1 avocado, cored, peeled, and roughly chopped	- lemon juice, 1½ lemons - ½ cup extra virgin olive oil - salt - pepper - 1 garlic clove, finely chopped - 2 tbsp fresh cilantro, finely chopped - 2 tbsp fresh mint, finely chopped	- Place the lemon-honey vinaigrette Ingredients: in a small bowl and whisk them well. - In a large mixing bowl, add baby arugula, fava beans, green onions, tomatoes, cucumbers, and jalapeno. - Divide the whole salad among four containers. - Before serving, dress the salad with the vinaigrette and toss. - Add the avocado to the salad. - Enjoy!

Chapter 4. DESSERTS

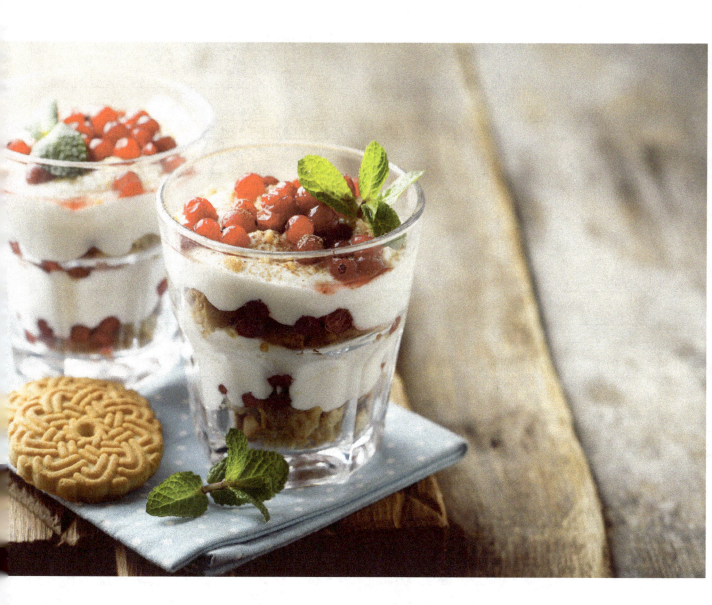

104) SOUTHERN AMERICAN APPLE COBBLER WITH RASPBERRIES

Preparation Time: 50 minutes

Servings: 4

Ingredients:
- 3 apples, chopped
- 2 tbsp pure date sugar
- 1 cup fresh raspberries
- 2 tbsp unsalted plant butter
- ½ cup whole-wheat flour
- 1 cup toasted rolled oats
- 2 tbsp pure date sugar
- 1 tsp cinnamon powder

Directions:
- Preheat the oven to 350 F and grease a baking dish with some plant butter.
- Add apples, date sugar, and 3 tbsp of water to a pot. Cook over low heat until the date sugar melts and then mix in the raspberries. Cook until the fruits soften, 10 minutes. Pour and spread the fruit mixture into the baking dish and set aside.
- In a blender, add the plant butter, flour, oats, date sugar, and cinnamon powder. Pulse a few times until crumbly. Spoon and spread the mixture on the fruit mix until evenly layered. Bake in the oven for 25 to 30 minutes or until golden brown on top. Remove the dessert, allow cooling for 2 minutes, and serve

105) SWEET CHOCOLATE PEPPERMINT MOUSSE

Preparation Time: 10 minutes + chilling time

Servings: 4

Ingredients:
- ¼ cup Swerve sugar, divided
- 4 oz cashew cream cheese, softened
- 3 tbsp cocoa powder
- ¾ tsp peppermint extract
- ½ tsp vanilla extract
- 1/3 cup coconut cream

Directions:
- Put 2 tbsp of Swerve sugar, cashew cream cheese, and cocoa powder in a blender. Add the peppermint extract, ¼ cup warm water, and process until smooth. In a bowl, whip vanilla extract, coconut cream, and the remaining Swerve sugar using a whisk. Fetch out 5-6 tbsp for garnishing. Fold in the cocoa mixture until thoroughly combined. Spoon the mousse into serving cups and chill in the fridge for 30 minutes. Garnish with the reserved whipped cream and serve

106) TASTY RASPBERRIES TURMERIC PANNA COTTA

Preparation Time: 10 minutes + chilling time

Servings: 6

Ingredients:
- ½ tbsp powdered vegetarian gelatin
- 2 cups coconut cream
- ¼ tsp vanilla extract
- 1 pinch turmeric powder
- 1 tbsp erythritol
- 1 tbsp chopped toasted pecans
- 12 fresh raspberries

Directions:
- Mix gelatin and ½ tsp water and allow sitting to dissolve. Pour coconut cream, vanilla extract, turmeric, and erythritol into a saucepan and bring to a boil over medium heat, then simmer for 2 minutes. Turn the heat off. Stir in the gelatin until dissolved. Pour the mixture into 6 glasses, cover with plastic wrap, and refrigerate for 2 hours or more. Top with the pecans and raspberries and serve

107) SPRING BANANA PUDDING

Preparation Time: 25 minutes + cooling time
Servings: 4

Ingredients:
- 1 cup unsweetened almond milk
- 2 cups cashew cream
- ¾ cup + 1 tbsp pure date sugar
- ¼ tsp salt
- 3 tbsp corn-starch
- 2 tbsp plant butter, cut into 4 pieces
- 1 tsp vanilla extract
- 2 banana, sliced

Directions:
- In a medium pot, mix almond milk, cashew cream, date sugar, and salt. Cook over medium heat until slightly thickened, 10-15 minutes. Stir in the corn-starch, plant butter, vanilla extract, and banana extract. Cook further for 1 to 2 minutes or until the pudding thickens. Dish the pudding into 4 serving bowls and chill in the refrigerator for at least 1 hour. To serve, top with the bananas and enjoy

108) EVERYDAY BAKED APPLES FILLED WITH NUTS

Preparation Time: 35 minutes + cooling time
Servings: 4

Ingredients:
- 4 gala apples
- 3 tbsp pure maple syrup
- 4 tbsp almond flour
- 6 tbsp pure date sugar
- 6 tbsp plant butter, cold and cubed
- 1 cup chopped mixed nuts

Directions:
- Preheat the oven the 400 F.
- Slice off the top of the apples and use a melon baller or spoon to scoop out the cores of the apples. In a bowl, mix the maple syrup, almond flour, date sugar, butter, and nuts. Spoon the mixture into the apples and then bake in the oven for 25 minutes or until the nuts are golden brown on top and the apples soft. Remove the apples from the oven, allow cooling, and serve

109) SUMMER MINT ICE CREAM

Preparation Time: 10 minutes + chilling time
Servings: 4

Ingredients:
- 2 avocados, pitted
- 1 ¼ cups coconut cream
- ½ tsp vanilla extract
- 2 tbsp erythritol
- 2 tsp chopped mint leaves

Directions:
- Into a blender, spoon the avocado pulps, pour in the coconut cream, vanilla extract, erythritol, and mint leaves. Process until smooth. Pour the mixture into your ice cream maker and freeze according to the manufacturer's instructions. When ready, remove and scoop the ice cream into bowls. Serve

110) TASTY CARDAMOM COCONUT FAT BOMBS

Preparation Time: 10 minutes
Servings: 6

Ingredients:
- ½ cup grated coconut
- 3 oz plant butter, softened
- ¼ tsp green cardamom powder
- ½ tsp vanilla extract
- ¼ tsp cinnamon powder

Directions:
- Pour the grated coconut into a skillet and roast until lightly brown. Set aside to cool. In a bowl, combine butter, half of the coconut, cardamom, vanilla, and cinnamon. Form balls from the mixture and roll each one in the remaining coconut. Refrigerate until ready to serve

111) HUNGARIAN CINNAMON FAUX RICE PUDDING

Preparation Time: 25 minutes | | **Servings:** 6

Ingredients:
- 1 ¼ cups coconut cream
- 1 tsp vanilla extract
- 1 tsp cinnamon powder
- 1 cup mashed tofu
- 2 oz fresh strawberries

Directions:
- Pour the coconut cream into a bowl and whisk until a soft peak forms. Mix in the vanilla and cinnamon. Lightly fold in the vegan cottage cheese and refrigerate for 10 to 15 minutes to set. Spoon into serving glasses, top with the strawberries and serve immediately

112) SWEET WHITE CHOCOLATE FUDGE

Preparation Time: 20 minutes + chilling time | | **Servings:** 6

Ingredients:
- 2 cups coconut cream
- 1 tsp vanilla extract
- 3 oz plant butter
- 3 oz vegan white chocolate
- Swerve sugar for sprinkling

Directions:
- Pour coconut cream and vanilla into a saucepan and bring to a boil over medium heat, then simmer until reduced by half, 15 minutes. Stir in plant butter until the batter is smooth. Chop white chocolate into bits and stir in the cream until melted. Pour the mixture into a baking sheet; chill in the fridge for 3 hours. Cut into squares, sprinkle with swerve sugar, and serve

113) ITALIAN MACEDONIA SALAD WITH COCONUT AND PECANS

Preparation Time: 15 minutes + cooling time | | **Servings:** 4

Ingredients:
- 1 cup pure coconut cream
- ½ tsp vanilla extract
- 2 bananas, cut into chunks
- 1 ½ cups coconut flakes
- 4 tbsp toasted pecans, chopped
- 1 cup pineapple tidbits, drained
- 1 (11-oz) can mandarin oranges
- ¾ cup maraschino cherries, stems removed

Directions:
- In a medium bowl, mix the coconut cream and vanilla extract until well combined.
- In a larger bowl, combine the bananas, coconut flakes, pecans, pineapple, oranges, and cherries until evenly distributed. Pour on the coconut cream mixture and fold well into the salad. Chill in the refrigerator for 1 hour and serve afterward

114) AUTHENTIC BERRY HAZELNUT TRIFLE

Preparation Time: 10 minutes | | **Servings:** 4

Ingredients:
- 1 ½ ripe avocados
- ¾ cup coconut cream
- Zest and juice of ½ a lemon
- 1 tbsp vanilla extract
- 3 oz fresh strawberries
- 2 oz toasted hazelnuts

Directions:
- In a bowl, add avocado pulp, coconut cream, lemon zest and juice, and half of the vanilla extract. Mix with an immersion blender. Put the strawberries and remaining vanilla in another bowl and use a fork to mash the fruits. In a tall glass, alternate layering the cream and strawberry mixtures. Drop a few hazelnuts on each and serve the dessert immediately

115) VEGETARIAN AVOCADO TRUFFLES WITH CHOCOLATE COATING

Preparation Time: 5 minutes

Servings: 6

Ingredients:
- 1 ripe avocado, pitted
- ½ tsp vanilla extract
- ½ tsp lemon zest
- 5 oz dairy-free dark chocolate
- 1 tbsp coconut oil
- 1 tbsp unsweetened cocoa powder

Directions:
- Scoop the pulp of the avocado into a bowl and mix with the vanilla using an immersion blender. Stir in the lemon zest and a pinch of salt. Pour the chocolate and coconut oil into a safe microwave bowl and melt in the microwave for 1 minute. Add to the avocado mixture and stir. Allow cooling to firm up a bit. Form balls out of the mix. Roll each ball in the cocoa powder and serve immediately

116) DELICIOUS VANILLA BERRY TARTS

Preparation Time: 35 minutes + cooling time

Servings: 4

Ingredients:
- 4 tbsp flaxseed powder
- 1/3 cup whole-wheat flour
- ½ tsp salt
- ¼ cup plant butter, crumbled
- 3 tbsp pure malt syrup
- 6 oz cashew cream
- 6 tbsp pure date sugar
- ¾ tsp vanilla extract
- 1 cup mixed frozen berries

Directions:
- Preheat oven to 350 F and grease mini pie pans with cooking spray. In a bowl, mix flaxseed powder with 12 tbsp water and allow soaking for 5 minutes. In a large bowl, combine flour and salt. Add in butter and whisk until crumbly. Pour in the vegan "flax egg" and malt syrup and mix until smooth dough forms. Flatten the dough on a flat surface, cover with plastic wrap, and refrigerate for 1 hour.
- Dust a working surface with some flour, remove the dough onto the surface, and using a rolling pin, flatten the dough into a 1-inch diameter circle. Use a large cookie cutter, cut out rounds of the dough and fit into the pie pans. Use a knife to trim the edges of the pan. Lay a parchment paper on the dough cups, pour on some baking beans, and bake in the oven until golden brown, 15-20 minutes. Remove the pans from the oven, pour out the baking beans, and allow cooling. In a bowl, mix cashew cream, date sugar, and vanilla extract. Divide the mixture into the tart cups and top with berries. Serve

117) BEST HOMEMADE CHOCOLATES WITH COCONUT AND RAISINS

Preparation Time: 10 minutes + chilling time

Servings: 20

Ingredients:
- 1/2 cup cacao butter, melted
- 1/3 cup peanut butter
- 1/4 cup agave syrup
- A pinch of grated nutmeg
- A pinch of coarse salt
- 1/2 tsp vanilla extract
- 1 cup dried coconut, shredded
- 6 ounces dark chocolate, chopped
- 3 ounces raisins

Directions:
- Thoroughly combine all the ingredients, except for the chocolate, in a mixing bowl.
- Spoon the mixture into molds. Leave to set hard in a cool place.
- Melt the dark chocolate in your microwave. Pour in the melted chocolate until the fillings are covered. Leave to set hard in a cool place.
- Enjoy

118) SIMPLE MOCHA FUDGE

Preparation Time: 1 hour 10 minutes

Servings: 20

Ingredients:
- 1 cup cookies, crushed
- 1/2 cup almond butter
- 1/4 cup agave nectar
- 6 ounces dark chocolate, broken into chunks
- 1 tsp instant coffee
- A pinch of grated nutmeg
- A pinch of salt

Directions:
- Line a large baking sheet with parchment paper.
- Melt the chocolate in your microwave and add in the remaining ingredients; stir to combine well.
- Scrape the batter into a parchment-lined baking sheet. Place it in your freezer for at least 1 hour to set.
- Cut into squares and serve. Enjoy

119) EAST ALMOND AND CHOCOLATE CHIP BARS

Preparation Time: 40 minutes

Servings: 10

Ingredients:
- 1/2 cup almond butter
- 1/4 cup coconut oil, melted
- 1/4 cup agave syrup
- 1 tsp vanilla extract
- 1/4 tsp sea salt
- 1/4 tsp grated nutmeg
- 1/2 tsp ground cinnamon
- 2 cups almond flour
- 1/4 cup flaxseed meal
- 1 cup vegan chocolate, cut into chunks
- 1 1/3 cups almonds, ground
- 2 tbsp cacao powder
- 1/4 cup agave syrup

Directions:
- In a mixing bowl, thoroughly combine the almond butter, coconut oil, 1/4 cup of agave syrup, vanilla, salt, nutmeg and cinnamon.
- Gradually stir in the almond flour and flaxseed meal and stir to combine. Add in the chocolate chunks and stir again.
- In a small mixing bowl, combine the almonds, cacao powder and agave syrup. Now, spread the ganache onto the cake. Freeze for about 30 minutes, cut into bars and serve well chilled. Enjoy

120) ALMOND BUTTER COOKIES

Preparation Time: 45 minutes

Servings: 10

Ingredients:
- 3/4 cup all-purpose flour
- 1/2 tsp baking soda
- 1/4 tsp kosher salt
- 1 flax egg
- 1/4 cup coconut oil, at room temperature
- 2 tbsp almond milk
- 1/2 cup brown sugar
- 1/2 cup almond butter
- 1/2 tsp ground cinnamon
- 1/2 tsp vanilla

Directions:
- In a mixing bowl, combine the flour, baking soda and salt.
- In another bowl, combine the flax egg, coconut oil, almond milk, sugar, almond butter, cinnamon and vanilla. Stir the wet mixture into the dry ingredients and stir until well combined.
- Place the batter in your refrigerator for about 30 minutes. Shape the batter into small cookies and arrange them on a parchment-lined cookie pan.
- Bake in the preheated oven at 350 degrees F for approximately 12 minutes. Transfer the pan to a wire rack to cool at room temperature. Enjoy

BOOK 2: THE PLANT-BASED DIET COOKBOOK

Chapter 1. BREAKFAST AND SNACKS

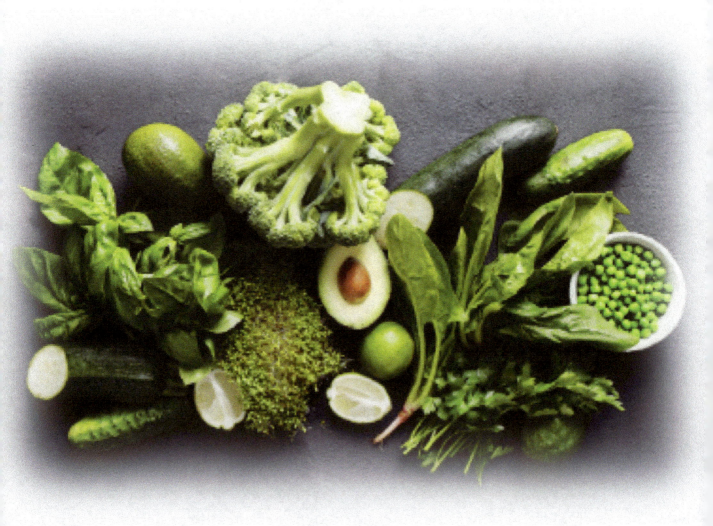

121) AMERICAN KENTUCKY CAULIFLOWER WITH MASHED PARSNIPS

Preparation Time: 35 minutes

Servings: 6

Ingredients:
- ½ cup unsweetened almond milk
- ¼ cup coconut flour
- ¼ tsp cayenne pepper
- ½ cup whole-grain breadcrumbs
- ½ cup grated plant-based mozzarella
- 30 oz cauliflower florets
- 1 lb parsnips, peeled and quartered
- 3 tbsp melted plant butter
- A pinch of nutmeg
- 1 tsp cumin powder
- 1 cup coconut cream
- 2 tbsp sesame oil

Directions:
- Preheat oven to 425 F and line a baking sheet with parchment paper.
- In a small bowl, combine almond milk, coconut flour, and cayenne pepper. In another bowl, mix salt, breadcrumbs, and plant-based mozzarella cheese. Dip each cauliflower floret into the milk mixture, coating properly, and then into the cheese mixture. Place the breaded cauliflower on the baking sheet and bake in the oven for 30 minutes, turning once after 15 minutes.
- Make slightly salted water in a saucepan and add the parsnips. Bring to boil over medium heat for 15 minutes or until the parsnips are fork-tender. Drain and transfer to a bowl. Add in melted plant butter, cumin powder, nutmeg, and coconut cream. Puree the ingredients using an immersion blender until smooth. Spoon the parsnip mash into serving plates and drizzle with some sesame oil. Serve with the baked cauliflower when ready

122) SPANISH SPINACH CHIPS WITH GUACAMOLE HUMMUS

Preparation Time: 30 minutes

Servings: 4

Ingredients:
- ½ cup baby spinach
- 1 tbsp olive oil
- ½ tsp plain vinegar
- 3 large avocados, chopped
- ½ cup chopped parsley + for garnish
- ½ cup melted plant butter
- ¼ cup pumpkin seeds
- ¼ cup sesame paste
- Juice from ½ lemon
- 1 garlic clove, minced
- ½ tsp coriander powder
- Salt and black pepper to taste

Directions:
- Preheat oven to 300 F. Put spinach in a bowl and toss with olive oil, vinegar, and salt. Place in a parchment paper-lined baking sheet and bake until the leaves are crispy but not burned, about 15 minutes.
- Place avocado into the bowl of a food processor. Add in parsley, plant butter, pumpkin seeds, sesame paste, lemon juice, garlic, coriander powder, salt, and black pepper. Puree until smooth. Spoon the hummus into a bowl and garnish with parsley. Serve with spinach chips

123) SUPER BUTTERED CARROT NOODLES WITH KALE

Preparation Time: 15 minutes

Servings: 4

Ingredients:
- 2 large carrots
- ¼ cup vegetable broth
- 4 tbsp plant butter
- 1 garlic clove, minced
- 1 cup chopped kale
- Salt and black pepper to taste

Directions:
- Peel the carrots with a slicer and run both through a spiralizer to form noodles.
- Pour the vegetable broth into a saucepan and add the carrot noodles. Simmer (over low heat) the carrots for 3 minutes. Strain through a colander and set the vegetables aside.
- Place a large skillet over medium heat and melt the plant butter. Add the garlic and sauté until softened and put in the kale; cook until wilted. Pour the carrots into the pan, season with salt and black pepper, and stir-fry for 3 to 4 minutes. Spoon the vegetables into a bowl and serve with pan-grilled tofu

124) HEALTHY PARSLEY PUMPKIN NOODLES

Preparation Time: 15 minutes

Servings: 4

- ¼ cup plant butter
- ½ cup chopped onion
- 1 lb pumpkin, spiralized
- 1 bunch kale, sliced
- ¼ cup chopped fresh parsley
- Salt and black pepper to taste

- Mel butter in a skillet over medium heat. Place the onion and cook for 3 minutes. Add in pumpkin and cook for another 7-8 minutes. Stir in kale and cook for another 2 minutes, until the kale wilts. Sprinkle with parsley, salt, and pepper and serve

125) EASY MIXED VEGETABLES WITH BASIL

Preparation Time: 40 minutes

Servings: 4

- 2 medium zucchinis, chopped
- 2 medium yellow squash, chopped
- 1 red onion, cut into 1-inch wedges
- 1 red bell pepper, diced
- 1 cup cherry tomatoes, halved
- 4 tbsp olive oil
- Salt and black pepper to taste
- 3 garlic cloves, minced
- 2/3 cup whole-wheat breadcrumbs
- 1 lemon, zested
- ¼ cup chopped fresh basil

- Preheat the oven to 450 F. Lightly grease a large baking sheet with cooking spray.
- In a medium bowl, add the zucchini, yellow squash, red onion, bell pepper, tomatoes, olive oil, salt, black pepper, and garlic. Toss well and spread the mixture on the baking sheet. Roast in the oven for 25 to 30 minutes or until the vegetables are tender while stirring every 5 minutes.
- Meanwhile, heat the olive oil in a medium skillet and sauté the garlic until fragrant. Mix in the breadcrumbs, lemon zest, and basil. Cook for 2 to 3 minutes. Remove the vegetables from the oven and toss in the breadcrumb's mixture. Serve

126) DELICIOUS ONION RINGS AND KALE DIP

Preparation Time: 35 minutes

Servings: 4

- 1 onion, sliced into rings
- 1 tbsp flaxseed meal + 3 tbsp water
- 1 cup almond flour
- ½ cup grated plant-based Parmesan
- 2 tsp garlic powder
- ½ tbsp sweet paprika powder
- 2 oz chopped kale
- 2 tbsp olive oil
- 2 tbsp dried cilantro
- 1 tbsp dried oregano
- Salt and black pepper to taste
- 1 cup tofu mayonnaise
- 4 tbsp coconut cream
- Juice of ½ a lemon

- Preheat oven to 400 F. In a bowl, mix the flaxseed meal and water and leave the mixture to thicken and fully absorb for 5 minutes. In another bowl, combine almond flour, plant-based Parmesan cheese, half of the garlic powder, sweet paprika, and salt. Line a baking sheet with parchment paper in readiness for the rings. When the vegan "flax egg" is ready, dip in the onion rings one after another, and then into the almond flour mixture. Place the rings on the baking sheet and grease with cooking spray. Bake for 15-20 minutes or until golden brown and crispy. Remove the onion rings into a serving bowl.
- Put kale in a food processor. Add in olive oil, cilantro, oregano, remaining garlic powder, salt, black pepper, tofu mayonnaise, coconut cream, and lemon juice; puree until nice and smooth. Allow the dip to sit for about 10 minutes for the flavors to develop. After, serve the dip with the crispy onion rings

127) PORTUGUESE SOY CHORIZO STUFFED CABBAGE ROLLS

Preparation Time: 35 minutes

Servings: 4

Ingredients:

- ¼ cup coconut oil, divided
- 1 large white onion, chopped
- 3 cloves garlic, minced, divided
- 1 cup crumbled soy chorizo
- 1 cup cauliflower rice
- 1 can tomato sauce
- 1 tsp dried oregano
- 1 tsp dried basil
- 8 full green cabbage leaves

- Heat half of the coconut oil in a saucepan over medium heat.
- Add half of the onion, half of the garlic, and all of the soy chorizo. Sauté for 5 minutes or until the chorizo has browned further, and the onion softened. Stir in the cauli rice, season with salt and black pepper, and cook for 3 to 4 minutes. Turn the heat off and set the pot aside.
- Heat the remaining oil in a saucepan over medium heat, add, and sauté the remaining onion and garlic until fragrant and soft. Pour in the tomato sauce, and season with salt, black pepper, oregano, and basil. Add ¼ cup water and simmer the sauce for 10 minutes.
- While the sauce cooks, lay the cabbage leaves on a flat surface and spoon the soy chorizo mixture into the middle of each leaf. Roll the leaves to secure the filling. Place the cabbage rolls in the tomato sauce and cook further for 10 minutes. When ready, serve the cabbage rolls with sauce over mashed broccoli or with mixed seed bread

128) ASIAN SESAME CABBAGE SAUTÉ

Preparation Time: 15 minutes

Servings: 4

Ingredients:
- 2 tbsp soy sauce
- 1 tbsp toasted sesame oil
- 1 tbsp hot sauce
- ½ tbsp pure date sugar
- ½ tbsp olive oil
- 1 head green cabbage, shredded
- 2 carrots, julienned
- 3 green onions, thinly sliced
- 2 garlic cloves, minced
- 1 tbsp fresh grated ginger
- Salt and black pepper to taste
- 1 tbsp sesame seeds

Directions:
- In a small bowl, mix the soy sauce, sesame oil, hot sauce, and date sugar.
- Heat the olive oil in a large skillet and sauté the cabbage, carrots, green onion, garlic, and ginger until softened, 5 minutes. Mix in the prepared sauce and toss well. Cook for 1 to 2 minutes. Dish the food and garnish with the sesame seeds

129) POMODORI STUFFED WITH CHICKPEAS AND QUINOA

Preparation Time: 50 minutes

Servings: 4

Ingredients:
- 8 medium tomatoes
- ¾ cup quinoa, rinsed and drained
- 1 ½ cups water
- 1 tbsp olive oil
- 1 small onion, diced
- 3 garlic cloves, minced
- 1 cup chopped spinach
- 1 (7 oz) can chickpeas, drained
- ½ cup chopped fresh basil

Directions:
- Preheat the oven to 400 F.
- Cut off the heads of tomatoes and use a paring knife to scoop the inner pulp of the tomatoes. Season with some olive oil, salt, and black pepper. Add the quinoa and water to a medium pot, season with salt, and cook until the quinoa is tender and the water absorbs, 10 to 15 minutes. Fluff and set aside.
- Heat the remaining olive oil in a skillet and sauté the onion and garlic for 30 seconds. Mix in the spinach and cook until wilted, 2 minutes. Stir in the basil, chickpeas, and quinoa; allow warming from 2 minutes.
- Spoon the mixture into the tomatoes, place the tomatoes into the baking dish and bake in the oven for 20 minutes or until the tomatoes soften. Remove the tomatoes from the oven and dish the food

130) HERBED VEGETABLE TRAYBAKE

Preparation Time: 85 minutes

Servings: 4

Ingredients:
- 2 tbsp plant butter
- 1 large onion, diced
- 1 cup celery, diced
- ½ cup carrots, diced
- ½ tsp dried marjoram
- 2 cups chopped cremini mushrooms
- 1 cup vegetable broth
- ¼ cup chopped fresh parsley
- 1 whole-grain bread loaf, cubed

Directions:
- Melt the butter in a large skillet and sauté onion, celery, mushrooms, and carrots for 5 minutes. Mix in marjoram, salt, and pepper. Pour in the vegetable broth and mix in parsley and bread. Cook until the broth reduces by half, 10 minutes. Pour the mixture into a baking dish and cover with foil. Bake in the oven at 375 F for 30 minutes. Uncover and bake further for 30 minutes or until golden brown on top, and the liquid absorbs. Remove the dish from the oven and serve the stuffing

131) AMERICAN LOUISIANA-STYLE SWEET POTATO CHIPS

Preparation Time: 55 minutes

Servings: 4

Ingredients:
- 2 sweet potatoes, peeled and sliced
- 2 tbsp melted plant butter
- 1 tbsp Cajun seasoning

Directions:
- Preheat the oven to 400 F and line a baking sheet with parchment paper.
- In a medium bowl, add the sweet potatoes, salt, plant butter, and Cajun seasoning. Toss well. Spread the chips on the baking sheet, making sure not to overlap, and bake in the oven for 50 minutes to 1 hour or until crispy. Remove the sheet and pour the chips into a large bowl. Allow cooling and enjoy

132) SPECIAL BELL PEPPER AND SEITAN BALLS

Preparation Time: 25 minutes **Servings:** 4

Ingredients:
- 1 tbsp flaxseed powder
- 1 lb seitan, crumbled
- ¼ cup chopped mixed bell peppers
- Salt and black pepper to taste
- 1 tbsp almond flour
- 1 tsp garlic powder
- 1 tsp onion powder
- 1 tsp tofu mayonnaise
- Olive oil for brushing

Directions:
- Preheat the oven to 400 F and line a baking sheet with parchment paper.
- In a bowl, mix flaxseed powder with 3 tbsp water and allow thickening for 5 minutes. Add in seitan, bell peppers, salt, pepper, almond flour, garlic powder, onion powder, and tofu mayonnaise. Mix and form 1-inch balls from the mixture. Arrange on the baking sheet, brush with cooking spray, and bake in the oven for 15 to 20 minutes or until brown and compacted. Remove from the oven and serve

133) ITALIAN PARMESAN BROCCOLI TOTS

Preparation Time: 30 minutes **Servings:** 4

Ingredients:
- 1 tbsp flaxseed powder
- 1 head broccoli, cut into florets
- 2/3 cup toasted almond flour
- 2 garlic cloves, minced
- 2 cups grated plant-based Parmesan
- Salt to taste

Directions:
- Preheat the oven to 350 F and line a baking sheet with parchment paper.
- In a small bowl, mix the flaxseed powder with the 3 tbsp water and allow thickening for 5 minutes to make the vegan "flax egg". Place the broccoli in a safe microwave bowl, sprinkle with 2 tbsp of water, and steam in the microwave for 1 minute or until softened. Transfer the broccoli to a food processor and add the vegan "flax egg," almond flour, garlic, plant cheese, and salt. Blend until coarsely smooth.
- Pour the mixture into a bowl and form 2-inch oblong balls from the mixture. Place the tots on the baking sheet and bake in the oven for 15 to 20 minutes or until firm and compacted. Remove the tots from the oven and serve warm with tomato dipping sauce.

134) TASTY CHOCOLATE BARS WITH WALNUTS

Preparation Time: 60 minutes **Servings:** 4

Ingredients:
- 1 cup walnuts
- 3 tbsp sunflower seeds
- 2 tbsp unsweetened chocolate chips
- 1 tbsp unsweetened cocoa powder
- 1 ½ tsp vanilla extract
- ¼ tsp cinnamon powder
- 2 tbsp melted coconut oil
- 2 tbsp toasted almond meal
- 2 tsp pure maple syrup

Directions:
- In a food processor, add the walnuts, sunflower seeds, chocolate chips, cocoa powder, vanilla extract, cinnamon powder, coconut oil, almond meal, maple syrup, and blitz a few times until combined.
- Line a flat baking sheet with plastic wrap, pour the mixture onto the sheet and place another plastic wrap on top. Use a rolling pin to flatten the batter and then remove the top plastic wrap. Freeze the snack until firm, 1 hour. Remove from the freezer, cut into 1 ½-inch sized bars and enjoy immediately

135) SIMPLE CARROT ENERGY BALLS

Preparation Time: 10 minutes + chilling time

Servings: 8

Ingredients:
- 1 large carrot, grated carrot
- 1 ½ cups old-fashioned oats
- 1 cup raisins
- 1 cup dates, pitied
- 1 cup coconut flakes
- 1/4 tsp ground cloves
- 1/2 tsp ground cinnamon

Directions:
- In your food processor, pulse all ingredients until it forms a sticky and uniform mixture.
- Shape the batter into equal balls.
- Place in your refrigerator until ready to serve. Enjoy

136) SUPER CRUNCHY SWEET POTATO BITES

Preparation Time: 25 minutes + chilling time

Servings: 4

Ingredients:
- 4 sweet potatoes, peeled and grated
- 2 chia eggs
- 1/4 cup nutritional yeast
- 2 tbsp tahini
- 2 tbsp chickpea flour
- 1 tsp shallot powder
- 1 tsp garlic powder
- 1 tsp paprika
- Sea salt and ground black pepper, to taste

Directions:
- Start by preheating your oven to 395 degrees F. Line a baking pan with parchment paper or Silpat mat.
- Thoroughly combine all the ingredients until everything is well incorporated.
- Roll the batter into equal balls and place them in your refrigerator for about 1 hour.
- Bake these balls for approximately 25 minutes, turning them over halfway through the cooking time. Enjoy

137) BEST ROASTED GLAZED BABY CARROTS

Preparation Time: 30 minutes

Servings: 6

Ingredients:
- 2 pounds baby carrots
- 1/4 cup olive oil
- 1/4 cup apple cider vinegar
- 1/2 tsp red pepper flakes
- Sea salt and freshly ground black pepper, to taste
- 1 tbsp agave syrup
- 2 tbsp soy sauce
- 1 tbsp fresh cilantro, minced

Directions:
- Start by preheating your oven 395 degrees F.
- Then, toss the carrots with the olive oil, vinegar, red pepper, salt, black pepper, agave syrup and soy sauce.
- Roast the carrots for about 30 minutes, rotating the pan once or twice. Garnish with fresh cilantro and serve. Enjoy

138) EVERYDAY OVEN-BAKED KALE CHIPS

Preparation Time: 20 minutes

Servings: 8

Ingredients:
- 2 bunches kale, leaves separated
- 2 tbsp olive oil
- 1/2 tsp mustard seeds
- 1/2 tsp celery seeds
- 1/2 tsp dried oregano
- 1/4 tsp ground cumin
- 1 tsp garlic powder
- Coarse sea salt and ground black pepper, to taste

Directions:
- Start by preheating your oven to 340 degrees F. Line a baking sheet with parchment paper or Silpat mar.
- Toss the kale leaves with the remaining ingredients until well coated.
- Bake in the preheated oven for about 13 minutes, rotating the pan once or twice. Enjoy

139) SPECIAL CHEESY CASHEW DIP

Preparation Time: 10 minutes

Servings: 8

Ingredients:
- 1 cup raw cashews
- 1 lemon, freshly squeezed
- 2 tbsp tahini
- 2 tbsp nutritional yeast
- 1/2 tsp turmeric powder
- 1/2 tsp red pepper flakes, crushed
- Sea salt and ground black pepper, to taste

Directions:
- Place all the ingredients in the bowl of your food processor. Blend until uniform, creamy and smooth. You can add a splash of water to thin it out, as needed.
- Spoon your dip into a serving bowl; serve with veggie sticks, chips, or crackers.
- Enjoy

140) HEALTHY PEPPERY HUMMUS DIP

Preparation Time: 10 minutes

Servings: 10

Ingredients:
- 20 ounces canned or boiled chickpeas, drained
- 1/4 cup tahini
- 2 garlic cloves, minced
- 2 tbsp lemon juice, freshly squeezed
- 1/2 cup chickpea liquid
- 2 red roasted peppers, seeded and sliced
- 1/2 tsp paprika
- 1 tsp dried basil
- Sea salt and ground black pepper, to taste
- 2 tbsp olive oil

Directions:
- Blitz all the ingredients, except for the oil, in your blender or food processor until your desired consistency is reached.
- Place in your refrigerator until ready to serve.
- Serve with toasted pita wedges or chips, if desired. Enjoy

141) ORIGINAL LEBANESE MUTABAL

Preparation Time: 10 minutes

Servings: 6

Ingredients:
- 1 pound eggplant
- 1 onion, chopped
- 1 tbsp garlic paste
- 4 tbsp tahini
- 1 tbsp coconut oil
- 2 tbsp lemon juice
- 1/2 tsp ground coriander
- 1/4 cup ground cloves
- 1 tsp red pepper flakes
- 1 tsp smoked peppers
- Sea salt and ground black pepper, to taste

Directions:
- Roast the eggplant until the skin turns black; peel the eggplant and transfer it to the bowl of your food processor.
- Add in the remaining ingredients. Blend until everything is well incorporated.
- Serve with crostini or pita bread, if desired. Enjoy

142) BEST INDIAN-STYLE ROASTED CHICKPEAS

Preparation Time: 10 minutes **Servings:** 8

Ingredients:
- 2 cups canned chickpeas, drained
- 2 tbsp olive oil
- 1/2 tsp garlic powder
- 1/2 tsp paprika
- 1 tsp curry powder
- 1 tsp garam masala
- Sea salt and red pepper, to taste

Directions:
- Pat the chickpeas dry using paper towels. Drizzle olive oil over the chickpeas.
- Roast the chickpeas in the preheated oven at 400 degrees F for about 25 minutes, tossing them once or twice.
- Toss your chickpeas with the spices and enjoy

143) EASY AVOCADO WITH TAHINI SAUCE

Preparation Time: 10 minutes **Servings:** 4

Ingredients:
- 2 large-sized avocados, pitted and halved
- 4 tbsp tahini
- 4 tbsp soy sauce
- 1 tbsp lemon juice
- 1/2 tsp red pepper flakes
- Sea salt and ground black pepper, to taste
- 1 tsp garlic powder

Directions:
- Place the avocado halves on a serving platter.
- Mix the tahini, soy sauce, lemon juice, red pepper, salt, black pepper and garlic powder in a small bowl. Divide the sauce between the avocado halves.
- Enjoy

144) HEALTHY SWEET POTATO TATER TOTS

Preparation Time: 25 minutes + chilling time **Servings:** 4

Ingredients:
- 1 ½ pounds sweet potatoes, grated
- 2 chia eggs
- 1/2 cup plain flour
- 1/2 cup breadcrumbs
- 3 tbsp hummus
- Sea salt and black pepper, to taste
- 1 tbsp olive oil
- 1/2 cup salsa sauce

Directions:
- Start by preheating your oven to 395 degrees F. Line a baking pan with parchment paper or Silpat mat.
- Thoroughly combine all the ingredients, except for the salsa, until everything is well incorporated.
- Roll the batter into equal balls and place them in your refrigerator for about 1 hour.
- Bake these balls for approximately 25 minutes, turning them over halfway through the cooking time. Enjoy

Chapter 2. LUNCH

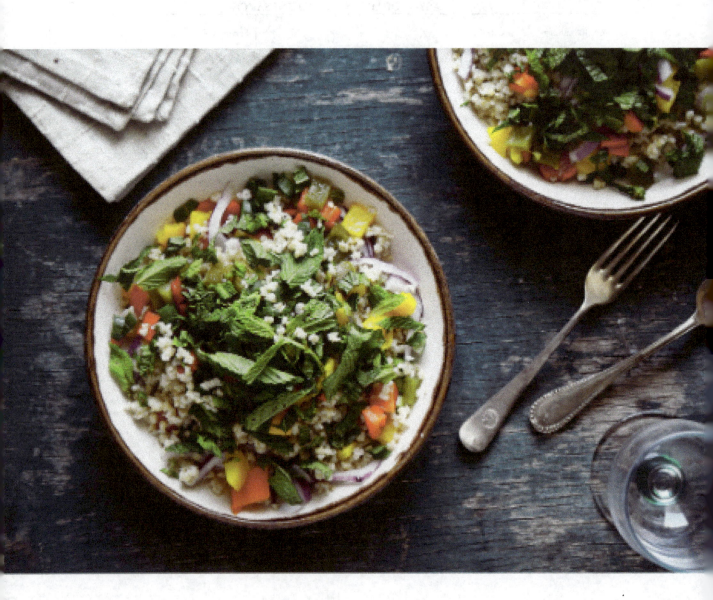

145) BEST BRAISED KALE WITH SESAME SEEDS

Preparation Time: 10 minutes **Servings:** 4

Ingredients:
- 1 cup vegetable broth
- 1 pound kale, cleaned, tough stems removed, torn into pieces
- 4 tbsp olive oil
- 6 garlic cloves, chopped
- 1 tsp paprika
- Kosher salt and ground black pepper, to taste
- 4 tbsp sesame seeds, lightly toasted

Directions:
- In a saucepan, bring the vegetable broth to a boil; add in the kale leaves and turn the heat to a simmer. Cook for about 5 minutes until kale has softened; reserve.
- Heat the oil in the same saucepan over medium heat. Once hot, sauté the garlic for about 30 seconds or until aromatic.
- Add in the reserved kale, paprika, salt and black pepper and let it cook for a few minutes more or until heated through.
- Garnish with lightly toasted sesame seeds and serve immediately. Enjoy

146) AUTUMN ROASTED VEGETABLES

Preparation Time: 45 minutes **Servings:** 4

Ingredients:
- 1/2 pound carrots, slice into 1-inch chunks
- 1/2 pound parsnips, slice into 1-inch chunks
- 1/2 pound celery, slice into 1-inch chunks
- 1/2 pound sweet potatoes, slice into 1-inch chunks
- 1 large onion, slice into wedges
- 1/4 cup olive oil
- 1 tsp red pepper flakes
- 1 tsp dried basil
- 1 tsp dried oregano
- 1 tsp dried thyme
- Sea salt and freshly ground black pepper

Directions:
- Start by preheating your oven to 420 degrees F.
- Toss the vegetables with the olive oil and spices. Arrange them on a parchment-lined roasting pan.
- Roast for about 25 minutes. Stir the vegetables and continue to cook for 20 minutes more.
- Enjoy!

147) AUTHENTIC MOROCCAN TAGINE

Preparation Time: 30 minutes **Servings:** 4

Ingredients:
- 3 tbsp olive oil
- 1 large shallot, chopped
- 1 tsp ginger, peeled and minced
- 4 garlic cloves, chopped
- 2 medium carrots, trimmed and chopped
- 2 medium parsnips, trimmed and chopped
- 2 medium sweet potatoes, peeled and cubed
- Sea salt and ground black pepper, to taste
- 1 tsp hot sauce
- 1 tsp fenugreek
- 1/2 tsp saffron
- 1/2 tsp caraway
- 2 large tomatoes, pureed
- 4 cups vegetable broth
- 1 lemon, cut into wedges

Directions:
- In a Dutch Oven, heat the olive oil over medium heat. Once hot, sauté the shallots for 4 to 5 minutes, until tender.
- Then, sauté the ginger and garlic for about 40 seconds or until aromatic.
- Add in the remaining ingredients, except for the lemon and bring to a boil. Immediately turn the heat to a simmer.
- Let it simmer for about 25 minutes or until the vegetables have softened. Serve with fresh lemon wedges and enjoy

148) CHINESE-STYLE CABBAGE STIR-FRY

Preparation Time: 10 minutes

Servings: 3

Ingredients:
- 3 tbsp sesame oil
- 1 pound Chinese cabbage, sliced
- 1/2 tsp Chinese five-spice powder
- Kosher salt, to taste
- 1/2 tsp Szechuan pepper
- 2 tbsp soy sauce
- 3 tbsp sesame seeds, lightly toasted

Directions:
- In a wok, heat the sesame oil until sizzling. Stir fry the cabbage for about 5 minutes.
- Stir in the spices and soy sauce and continue to cook, stirring frequently, for about 5 minutes more, until the cabbage is crisp-tender and aromatic.
- Sprinkle sesame seeds over the top and serve immediately

149) SPECIAL SAUTÉED CAULIFLOWER WITH SESAME SEEDS

Preparation Time: 15 minutes

Servings: 4

Ingredients:
- 1 cup vegetable broth
- 1 ½ pounds cauliflower florets
- 4 tbsp olive oil
- 2 scallion stalks, chopped
- 4 garlic cloves, minced
- Sea salt and freshly ground black pepper, to taste
- 2 tbsp sesame seeds, lightly toasted

Directions:
- In a large saucepan, bring the vegetable broth to a boil; then, add in the cauliflower and cook for about 6 minutes or until fork-tender; reserve.
- Then, heat the olive oil until sizzling; now, sauté the scallions and garlic for about 1 minute or until tender and aromatic.
- Add in the reserved cauliflower, followed by salt and black pepper; continue to simmer for about 5 minutes or until heated through
- Garnish with toasted sesame seeds and serve immediately. Enjoy

150) BEST SWEET MASHED CARROTS

Preparation Time: 25 minutes

Servings: 4

Ingredients:
- 1 ½ pounds carrots, trimmed
- 3 tbsp vegan butter
- 1 cup scallions, sliced
- 1 tbsp maple syrup
- 1/2 tsp garlic powder
- 1/2 tsp ground allspice
- Sea salt, to taste
- 1/2 cup soy sauce
- 2 tbsp fresh cilantro, chopped

Directions:
- Steam the carrots for about 15 minutes until they are very tender; drain well.
- In a sauté pan, melt the butter until sizzling. Now, turn the heat down to maintain an insistent sizzle.
- Now, cook the scallions until they've softened. Add in the maple syrup, garlic powder, ground allspice, salt and soy sauce for about 10 minutes or until they are caramelized.
- Add the caramelized scallions to your food processor; add in the carrots and puree the ingredients until everything is well blended.
- Serve garnished with the fresh cilantro. Enjoy

151) LOVELY SAUTÉED TURNIP GREENS

Preparation Time: 15 minutes

Servings: 4

Ingredients:
- 2 tbsp olive oil
- 1 onion, sliced
- 2 garlic cloves, sliced
- 1 ½ pounds turnip greens cleaned and chopped
- 1/4 cup vegetable broth
- 1/4 cup dry white wine
- 1/2 tsp dried oregano
- 1 tsp dried parsley flakes
- Kosher salt and ground black pepper, to taste

Directions:
- In a sauté pan, heat the olive oil over a moderately high heat.
- Now, sauté the onion for 3 to 4 minutes or until tender and translucent. Add in the garlic and continue to cook for 30 seconds more or until aromatic.
- Stir in the turnip greens, broth, wine, oregano and parsley; continue sautéing an additional 6 minutes or until they have wilted completely.
- Season with salt and black pepper to taste and serve warm. Enjoy

152) ASIAN YUKON GOLD MASHED POTATOES

Preparation Time: 25 minutes — **Servings:** 5

Ingredients:
- 2 pounds Yukon Gold potatoes, peeled and diced
- 1 clove garlic, pressed
- Sea salt and red pepper flakes, to taste
- 3 tbsp vegan butter
- 1/2 cup soy milk
- 2 tbsp scallions, sliced

Directions:
- Cover the potatoes with an inch or two of cold water. Cook the potatoes in gently boiling water for about 20 minutes.
- Then, puree the potatoes, along with the garlic, salt, red pepper, butter and milk, to your desired consistency.
- Serve garnished with fresh scallions. Enjoy

153) SUPER AROMATIC SAUTÉED SWISS CHARD

Preparation Time: 15 minutes — **Servings:** 4

Ingredients:
- 2 tbsp vegan butter
- 1 onion, chopped
- 2 cloves garlic, sliced
- Sea salt and ground black pepper, to season
- 1 ½ pounds Swiss chard, torn into pieces, tough stalks removed
- 1 cup vegetable broth
- 1 bay leaf
- 1 thyme sprig
- 2 rosemary sprigs
- 1/2 tsp mustard seeds
- 1 tsp celery seeds

Directions:
- In a saucepan, melt the vegan butter over medium-high heat.
- Then, sauté the onion for about 3 minutes or until tender and translucent; sauté the garlic for about 1 minute until aromatic.
- Add in the remaining ingredients and turn the heat to a simmer; let it simmer, covered, for about 10 minutes or until everything is cooked through. Enjoy

154) TYPICAL SAUTÉED BELL PEPPERS

Preparation Time: 15 minutes — **Servings:** 2

Ingredients:
- 3 tbsp olive oil
- 4 bell peppers, seeded and slice into strips
- 2 cloves garlic, minced
- Salt and freshly ground black pepper, to taste
- 1 tsp cayenne pepper
- 4 tbsp dry white wine
- 2 tbsp fresh cilantro, roughly chopped

Directions:
- In a saucepan, heat the oil over medium-high heat.
- Once hot, sauté the peppers for about 4 minutes or until tender and fragrant. Then, sauté the garlic for about 1 minute until aromatic.
- Add in the salt, black pepper and cayenne pepper; continue to sauté, adding the wine, for about 6 minutes more until tender and cooked through.
- Taste and adjust the seasonings. Top with fresh cilantro and serve. Enjoy

155) CLASSIC MASHED ROOT VEGETABLES

Preparation Time: 25 minutes — **Servings:** 5

Ingredients:
- 1 pound russet potatoes, peeled and cut into chunks
- 1/2 pound parsnips, trimmed and diced
- 1/2 pound carrots, trimmed and diced
- 4 tbsp vegan butter
- 1 tsp dried oregano
- 1/2 tsp dried dill weed
- 1/2 tsp dried marjoram
- 1 tsp dried basil

Directions:
- Cover the vegetables with the water by 1 inch. Bring to a boil and cook for about 25 minutes until they've softened; drain.
- Mash the vegetables with the remaining ingredients, adding cooking liquid, as needed.
- Serve warm and enjoy

156) EASY ROASTED BUTTERNUT SQUASH

Preparation Time: 25 minutes

Servings: 4

Ingredients:
- 4 tbsp olive oil
- 1/2 tsp ground cumin
- 1/2 tsp ground allspice
- 1 ½ pounds butternut squash, peeled, seeded and diced
- 1/4 cup dry white wine
- 2 tbsp dark soy sauce
- 1 tsp mustard seeds
- 1 tsp paprika
- Sea salt and ground black pepper, to taste

Directions:
- Start by preheating your oven to 420 degrees F. Toss the squash with the remaining ingredients.
- Roast the butternut squash for about 25 minutes or until tender and caramelized.
- Serve warm and enjoy

157) CLASSICAL SAUTÉED CREMINI MUSHROOMS

Preparation Time: 10 minutes

Servings: 4

Ingredients:
- 4 tbsp olive oil
- 4 tbsp shallots, chopped
- 2 cloves garlic, minced
- 1 ½ pounds Cremini mushrooms, sliced
- 1/4 cup dry white wine
- Sea salt and ground black pepper, to taste

Directions:
- In a sauté pan, heat the olive oil over a moderately high heat.
- Now, sauté the shallot for 3 to 4 minutes or until tender and translucent. Add in the garlic and continue to cook for 30 seconds more or until aromatic.
- Stir in the Cremini mushrooms, wine, salt and black pepper; continue sautéing an additional 6 minutes, until your mushrooms are lightly browned.
- Enjoy

158) EASY ROASTED ASPARAGUS WITH SESAME SEEDS

Preparation Time: 25 minutes

Servings: 4

Ingredients:
- 1 ½ pounds asparagus, trimmed
- 4 tbsp extra-virgin olive oil
- Sea salt and ground black pepper, to taste
- 1/2 tsp dried oregano
- 1/2 tsp dried basil
- 1 tsp red pepper flakes, crushed
- 4 tbsp sesame seeds
- 2 tbsp fresh chives, roughly chopped

Directions:
- Start by preheating the oven to 400 degrees F. Then, line a baking sheet with parchment paper.
- Toss the asparagus with the olive oil, salt, black pepper, oregano, basil and red pepper flakes. Now, arrange your asparagus in a single layer on the prepared baking sheet.
- Roast your asparagus for approximately 20 minutes.
- Sprinkle sesame seeds over your asparagus and continue to bake an additional 5 minutes or until the asparagus spears are crisp-tender and the sesame seeds are lightly toasted.
- Garnish with fresh chives and serve warm. Enjoy

159) SPECIAL GREEK-STYLE EGGPLANT SKILLET

Preparation Time: 15 minutes

Servings: 4

Ingredients:
- 4 tbsp olive oil
- 1 ½ pounds eggplant, peeled and sliced
- 1 tsp garlic, minced
- 1 tomato, crushed
- Sea salt and ground black pepper, to taste
- 1 tsp cayenne pepper
- 1/2 tsp dried oregano
- 1/4 tsp ground bay leaf
- 2 ounces Kalamata olives, pitted and sliced

Directions:
- Heat the oil in a sauté pan over medium-high flame.
- Then, sauté the eggplant for about 9 minutes or until just tender.
- Add in the remaining ingredients, cover and continue to cook for 2 to 3 minutes more or until thoroughly cooked. Serve warm

160) SIMPLE CAULIFLOWER RICE

Preparation Time: 10 minutes   **Servings:** 5

Ingredients:
- 2 medium heads cauliflower, stems and leaves removed
- 4 tbsp extra-virgin olive oil
- 4 garlic cloves, pressed
- 1/2 tsp red pepper flakes, crushed
- Sea salt and ground black pepper, to taste
- 1/4 cup flat-leaf parsley, roughly chopped

Directions:
- Pulse the cauliflower in a food processor with the S-blade until they're broken into "rice".
- Heat the olive oil in a saucepan over medium-high heat. Once hot, cook the garlic until fragrant or about 1 minute.
- Add in the cauliflower rice, red pepper, salt and black pepper and continue sautéing for a further 7 to 8 minutes.
- Taste, adjust the seasonings and garnish with fresh parsley. Enjoy

161) SIMPLE GARLICKY KALE

Preparation Time: 10 minutes   **Servings:** 4

Ingredients:
- 4 tbsp olive oil
- 4 cloves garlic, chopped
- 1 ½ pounds fresh kale, tough stems and ribs removed, torn into pieces
- 1 cup vegetable broth
- 1/2 tsp cumin seeds
- 1/2 tsp dried oregano
- 1/2 tsp paprika
- 1 tsp onion powder
- Sea salt and ground black pepper, to taste

Directions:
- In a saucepan, heat the olive oil over a moderately high heat. Now, sauté the garlic for about 1 minute or until aromatic.
- Add in the kale in batches, gradually adding the vegetable broth; stir to promote even cooking.
- Turn the heat to a simmer, add in the spices and let it cook for 5 to 6 minutes, until the kale leaves wilt.
- Serve warm and enjoy

162) VEGETARIAN TOFU CABBAGE STIR-FRY

Preparation Time: 45 minutes   **Servings:** 4

Ingredients:
- 2 ½ cups baby bok choy, quartered
- 5 oz plant butter
- 2 cups tofu, cubed
- 1 tsp garlic powder
- 1 tsp onion powder
- 1 tbsp plain vinegar
- 2 garlic cloves, minced
- 1 tsp chili flakes
- 1 tbsp fresh ginger, grated
- 3 green onions, sliced
- 1 tbsp sesame oil
- 1 cup tofu mayonnaise

Directions:
- Melt half of the butter in a wok over medium heat, add the bok choy, and stir-fry until softened. Season with salt, black pepper, garlic powder, onion powder, and plain vinegar. Sauté for 2 minutes; set aside. Melt the remaining butter in the wok, add and sauté garlic, chili flakes, and ginger until fragrant. Put the tofu in the wok and cook until browned on all sides. Add the green onions and bok choy, heat for 2 minutes, and add the sesame oil. Stir in tofu mayonnaise, cook for 1 minute, and serve

163) SPECIAL SMOKED TEMPEH WITH BROCCOLI FRITTERS

Preparation Time: 40 minutes   **Servings:** 4

Ingredients:
- 4 tbsp flax seed powder
- 1 tbsp soy sauce
- 3 tbsp olive oil
- 1 tbsp grated ginger
- 3 tbsp fresh lime juice
- Cayenne pepper to taste
- 10 oz tempeh slices
- 1 head broccoli, grated
- 8 oz tofu, grated
- 3 tbsp almond flour
- ½ tsp onion powder
- 4 ¼ oz plant butter
- ½ cup mixed salad greens
- 1 cup tofu mayonnaise
- Juice of ½ a lemon

Directions:
- In a bowl, mix the flax seed powder with 12 tbsp water and set aside to soak for 5 minutes. In another bowl, combine soy sauce, olive oil, grated ginger, lime juice, salt, and cayenne pepper. Brush the tempeh slices with the mixture. Heat a grill pan over medium and grill the tempeh on both sides until golden brown and nicely smoked. Remove the slices to a plate.
- In another bowl, mix the tofu with broccoli. Add in vegan "flax egg," almond flour, onion powder, salt, and black pepper. Mix and form 12 patties out of the mixture. Melt the plant butter in a skillet and fry the patties on both sides until golden brown. Remove to a plate. Add the grilled tempeh with the broccoli fritters and salad greens. Mix the tofu mayonnaise with the lemon juice and drizzle over the salad

164) SIMPLE CHEESY CAULIFLOWER CASSEROLE

Preparation Time: 35 minutes | | **Servings:** 4

Ingredients:
- 2 oz plant butter
- 1 white onion, finely chopped
- ½ cup celery stalks, finely chopped
- 1 green bell pepper, chopped
- Salt and black pepper to taste
- 1 small head cauliflower, chopped
- 1 cup tofu mayonnaise
- 4 oz grated plant-based Parmesan
- 1 tsp red chili flakes

Directions:
- Preheat oven to 400 F. Season onion, celery, and bell pepper with salt and black pepper. In a bowl, mix cauliflower, tofu mayonnaise, Parmesan cheese, and red chili flakes. Pour the mixture into a greased baking dish and add the vegetables; mix to distribute. Bake for 20 minutes. Remove and serve warm

165) VERY SPICY VEGGIE STEAKS WITH GREEN SALAD

Preparation Time: 35 minutes | | **Servings:** 2

Ingredients:
- 1 eggplant, sliced
- 1 zucchini, sliced
- ¼ cup coconut oil
- Juice of ½ a lemon
- 5 oz plant-based cheddar, cubed
- 10 Kalamata olives
- 2 tbsp pecans
- 1 oz mixed salad greens
- ½ cup tofu mayonnaise
- Salt to taste
- ½ tsp Cayenne pepper to taste

Directions:
- Set oven to broil and line a baking sheet with parchment paper. Arrange eggplant and zucchini on the baking sheet. Brush with coconut oil and sprinkle with cayenne pepper. Broil for 15-20 minutes.
- Remove to a serving platter and drizzle with the lemon juice. Arrange the plant-based cheddar cheese, Kalamata olives, pecans, and mixed greens with the grilled veggies. Top with tofu mayonnaise and serve

166) MEXICAN-STYLE JALAPEÑO QUINOA BOWL WITH LIMA BEANS

Preparation Time: 30 minutes | | **Servings:** 4

Ingredients:
- 1 tbsp olive oil
- 1 lb extra firm tofu, cubed
- Salt and black pepper to taste
- 1 medium yellow onion, finely diced
- ½ cup cauliflower florets
- 1 jalapeño pepper, minced
- 2 garlic cloves, minced
- 1 tbsp red chili powder
- 1 tsp cumin powder
- 1 (8 oz) can sweet corn kernels
- 1 (8 oz) can lima beans, rinsed
- 1 cup quick-cooking quinoa
- 1 (14 oz) can diced tomatoes
- 2 ½ cups vegetable broth
- 1 cup grated plant-based cheddar
- 2 tbsp chopped fresh cilantro
- 2 limes, cut into wedges
- 1 avocado, pitted, sliced, and peeled

Directions:
- Heat olive oil in a pot and cook the tofu until golden brown, 5 minutes. Season with salt, pepper, and mix in onion, cauliflower, and jalapeño pepper. Cook until the vegetables soften, 3 minutes.
- Stir in garlic, chili powder, and cumin powder; cook for 1 minute. Mix in sweet corn kernels, lima beans, quinoa, tomatoes, and vegetable broth. Simmer until the quinoa absorbs all the liquid, 10 minutes. Fluff quinoa. Top with the plant-based cheddar cheese, cilantro, lime wedges, and avocado. Serve

167) ITAIAN BLACK-EYED PEA OAT BAKE

Preparation Time: 25 minutes | | **Servings:** 4

Ingredients:
- 1 carrot, shredded
- 1 onion, chopped
- 2 garlic cloves, minced
- 1 (15.5-oz) can black-eyed peas
- ¾ cup whole-wheat flour
- ¾ cup quick-cooking oats
- ½ cup breadcrumbs
- ¼ cup minced fresh parsley
- 1 tbsp soy sauce
- ½ tsp dried sage
- Salt and black pepper to taste

Directions:
- Preheat oven to 360 F.
- Combine the carrot, onion, garlic, and peas and pulse until creamy and smooth in a blender. Add in flour, oats, breadcrumbs, parsley, soy sauce, sage, salt, and pepper. Blend until ingredients are evenly mixed. Spoon the mixture into a greased loaf pan. Bake for 40 minutes until golden. Allow it to cool down for a few minutes before slicing. Serve immediately

168) HUNGARIAN PAPRIKA FAVA BEAN PATTIES

Preparation Time: 15 minutes **Servings:** 4

Ingredients:
- 4 tbsp olive oil
- 1 minced onion
- 1 garlic clove, minced
- 1 (15.5-oz) can fava beans
- 1 tbsp minced fresh parsley
- ½ cup breadcrumbs
- ¼ cup almond flour
- 1 tsp smoked paprika
- ½ tsp dried thyme
- 4 burger buns, toasted
- 4 lettuce leaves
- 1 ripe tomato, sliced

Directions:
- In a blender, add onion, garlic, beans, parsley, breadcrumbs, flour, paprika, thyme, salt, and pepper. Pulse until uniform but not smooth. Shape 4 patties out of the mixture. Refrigerate for 15 minutes.
- Heat olive oil in a skillet over medium heat. Fry the patties for 10 minutes on both sides until golden brown. Serve in toasted buns with lettuce and tomato slices

169) SIMPLE WALNUT LENTIL BURGERS

Preparation Time: 70 minutes **Servings:** 4

Ingredients:
- 2 tbsp olive oil
- 1 cup dry lentils, rinsed
- 2 carrots, grated
- 1 onion, diced
- ½ cup walnuts
- 1 tbsp tomato puree
- ¾ cup almond flour
- 2 tsp curry powder
- 4 whole-grain buns

Directions:
- Place lentils in a pot and cover with water. Bring to a boil and simmer for 15-20 minutes.
- Meanwhile, combine the carrots, walnuts, onion, tomato puree, flour, curry powder, salt, and pepper in a bowl. Toss to coat. Once the lentils are ready, drain and transfer into the veggie bowl. Mash the mixture until sticky. Shape the mixture into balls; flatten to make patties.
- Heat the oil in a skillet over medium heat. Brown the patties for 8 minutes on both sides. To assemble, put the cakes on the buns and top with your desired toppings

170) ASIAN COUSCOUS ANDQUINOA BURGERS

Preparation Time: 20 minutes **Servings:** 4

Ingredients:
- 2 tbsp olive oil
- ¼ cup couscous
- ¼ cup boiling water
- 2 cups cooked quinoa
- 2 tbsp balsamic vinegar
- 3 tbsp chopped olives
- ½ tsp garlic powder
- Salt to taste
- 4 burger buns
- Lettuce leaves, for serving
- Tomato slices, for serving

Directions:
- Preheat oven to 350 F.
- In a bowl, place the couscous with boiling water. Let sit covered for 5 minutes. Once the liquid is absorbed, fluff with a fork. Add in quinoa and mash them to form a chunky texture. Stir in vinegar, olive oil, olives, garlic powder, and salt.
- Shape the mixture into 4 patties. Arrange them on a greased tray and bake for 25-30 minutes. To assemble, place the patties on the buns and top with lettuce and tomato slices. Serve

171) SPECIAL BEAN AND PECAN SANDWICHES

Preparation Time: 20 minutes **Servings:** 4

Ingredients:
- 1 onion, chopped
- 1 garlic clove, crushed
- ¾ cup pecans, chopped
- ¾ cup canned black beans
- ¾ cup almond flour
- 2 tbsp minced fresh parsley
- 1 tbsp soy sauce
- 1 tsp Dijon mustard + to serve
- Salt and black pepper to taste
- ½ tsp ground sage
- ½ tsp sweet paprika
- 2 tbsp olive oil
- Bread slices
- Lettuce leaves and sliced tomatoes

Directions:
- Put the onion, garlic, and pecans in a blender and pulse until roughly ground. Add in the beans and pulse until everything is well combined. Transfer to a large mixing bowl and stir in the flour, parsley, soy sauce, mustard, salt, sage, paprika, and pepper. Mold patties out of the mixture.
- Heat the oil in a skillet over medium heat. Brown the patties for 10 minutes on both sides. To assemble, lay patties on the bread slices and top with mustard, lettuce, and tomato slices

172) SIMPLE HOMEMADE KITCHARI

Preparation Time: 40 minutes **Servings:** 5

Ingredients:
- 4 cups chopped cauliflower and broccoli florets
- ½ cup split peas
- ½ cup brown rice
- 1 red onion, chopped
- 1 (14.5-oz) can diced tomatoes
- 3 garlic cloves, minced
- 1 jalapeño pepper, seeded
- ½ tsp ground ginger
- 1 tsp ground turmeric
- 1 tsp olive oil
- 1 tsp fennel seeds
- Juice of 1 large lemon
- Salt and black pepper to taste

Directions:
- In a food processor, place the onion, tomatoes with juices, garlic, jalapeño pepper, ginger, turmeric, and 2 tbsp of water. Pulse until ingredients are evenly mixed.
- Heat the oil in a pot over medium heat. Cook the cumin and fennel seeds for 2-3 minutes, stirring often. Pour in the puréed mixture, split peas, rice, and 3 cups of water. Bring to a boil, then lower the heat and simmer for 10 minutes. Stir in cauliflower, broccoli, and cook for another 10 minutes. Mix in lemon juice and adjust seasoning

173) PICCANTE GREEN RICE

Preparation Time: 35 minutes **Servings:** 4

Ingredients:
- 1 roasted bell pepper, chopped
- 3 small hot green chilies, chopped
- 2 ½ cups vegetable broth
- ½ cup chopped fresh parsley
- 1 onion, chopped
- 2 garlic cloves, chopped
- Salt and black pepper to taste
- ½ tsp dried oregano
- 3 tbsp canola oil
- 1 cup long-grain brown rice
- 1 ½ cups cooked black beans
- 2 tbsp minced fresh cilantro

Directions:
- In a food processor, place bell pepper, chilies, 1 cup of broth, parsley, onion, garlic, pepper, oregano, salt, and pepper and blend until smooth. Heat oil in a skillet over medium heat. Add in rice and veggie mixture. Cook for 5 minutes, stirring often. Add in the remaining broth and bring to a boil, lower the heat, and simmer for 15 minutes. Mix in beans and cook for another 5 minutes. Serve with cilantro

174) SPECIAL ASIAN QUINOA SAUTÉ

Preparation Time: 30 minutes **Servings:** 4

Ingredients:
- 1 cup quinoa
- Salt to taste
- 1 head cauliflower, break into florets
- 2 tsp untoasted sesame oil
- 1 cup snow peas, cut in half
- 1 cup frozen peas
- 2 cups chopped Swiss chard
- 2 scallions, chopped
- 2 tbsp water
- 1 tsp toasted sesame oil
- 1 tbsp soy sauce
- 2 tbsp sesame seeds

Directions:
- Place quinoa with 2 cups of water and salt in a bowl. Bring to a boil, lower the heat and simmer for 15 minutes. Do not stir.
- Heat the oil in a skillet over medium heat and sauté the cauliflower for 4-5 minutes. Add in snow peas and stir well. Stir in Swiss chard, scallions, and 2 tbsp of water; cook until wilted, about 5 minutes. Season with salt.
- Drizzle with sesame oil and soy sauce and cook for 1 minute. Divide the quinoa in bowls and top with the cauliflower mixture. Garnish with sesame seeds and soy sauce to serve

175) ITALIAN FARRO AND BLACK BEAN LOAF

Preparation Time: 50 minutes **Servings:** 6

Ingredients:
- 3 tbsp olive oil
- 1 onion, minced
- 1 cup faro
- 2 (15.5-oz) cans black beans, mashed
- ½ cup quick-cooking oats
- 1/3 cup whole-wheat flour
- 2 tbsp nutritional yeast
- 1 ½ tsp dried thyme
- ½ tsp dried oregano

Directions:
- Heat the oil in a pot over medium heat. Place in onion and sauté for 3 minutes. Add in faro, 2 cups of water, salt, and pepper. Bring to a boil, lower the heat and simmer for 20 minutes. Remove to a bowl.
- Preheat oven to 350 F.
- Add the mashed beans, oats, flour, yeast, thyme, and oregano to the faro bowl. Toss to combine. Taste and adjust the seasoning. Shape the mixture into a greased loaf. Bake for 20 minutes. Let cool for a few minutes. Slice and serve

176) SPECIAL CUBAN-STYLE MILLET

Preparation Time: 40 minutes   **Servings:** 4

Ingredients:
- 2 tbsp olive oil
- 1 onion, chopped
- 2 zucchinis, chopped
- 2 garlic cloves, minced
- 1 tsp dried thyme
- ½ tsp ground cumin
- 1 (15.5-oz) can black-eyed peas
- 1 cup millet
- 2 tbsp chopped fresh cilantro

Directions:
- Heat the oil in a pot over medium heat. Place in onion and sauté for 3 minutes until translucent. Add in zucchinis, garlic, thyme, and cumin and cook for 10 minutes. Put in peas, millet, and 2 ½ cups of hot water. Bring to a boil, then lower the heat and simmer for 20 minutes. Fluff the millet using a fork. Serve garnished with cilantro

177) CLASSIC CILANTRO PILAF

Preparation Time: 30 minutes   **Servings:** 6

Ingredients:
- 3 tbsp olive oil
- 1 onion, minced
- 1 carrot, chopped
- 2 garlic cloves, minced
- 1 cup wild rice
- 1 ½ tsp ground fennel seeds
- ½ tsp ground cumin
- Salt and black pepper to taste
- 3 tbsp minced fresh cilantro

Directions:
- Heat the oil in a pot over medium heat. Place in onion, carrot, and garlic and sauté for 5 minutes. Stir in rice, fennel seeds, cumin, and 2 cups water. Bring to a boil, then lower the heat and simmer for 20 minutes. Remove to a bowl and fluff using a fork. Serve topped with cilantro and black pepper

178) TYPICAL ORIENTAL BULGUR AND WHITE BEANS

Preparation Time: 55 minutes   **Servings:** 4

Ingredients:
- 2 tbsp olive oil
- 3 green onions, chopped
- 1 cup bulgur
- 1 cups water
- 1 tbsp soy sauce
- Salt to taste
- 1 ½ cups cooked white beans
- 1 tbsp nutritional yeast
- 1 tbsp dried parsley

Directions:
- Heat the oil in a pot over medium heat. Place in green onions and sauté for 3 minutes. Stir in bulgur, water, soy sauce, and salt. Bring to a boil, then lower the heat and simmer for 20-22 minutes. Mix in beans and yeast. Cook for 5 minutes. Serve topped with parsley

179) RED LENTILS WITH MUSHROOMS

Preparation Time: 25 minutes   **Servings:** 4

Ingredients:
- 2 tsp olive oil
- 2 cloves garlic, minced
- 2 tsp grated fresh ginger
- ½ tsp ground cumin
- ½ tsp fennel seeds
- 1 cup mushrooms, chopped
- 1 large tomato, chopped
- 1 cup dried red lentils
- 2 tbsp lemon juice

Directions:
- Heat the oil in a pot over medium heat. Place in the garlic and ginger and cook for 3 minutes. Stir in cumin, fennel, mushrooms, tomato, lentils, and 2 ¼ cups of water. Bring to a boil, then lower the heat and simmer for 15 minutes. Mix in lemon juice and serve

180) SPECIAL COLORFUL RISOTTO WITH VEGETABLES

Preparation Time: 35 minutes

Servings: 5

Ingredients:
- 2 tbsp sesame oil
- 1 onion, chopped
- 2 bell peppers, chopped
- 1 parsnip, trimmed and chopped
- 1 carrot, trimmed and chopped
- 1 cup broccoli florets
- 2 garlic cloves, finely chopped
- 1/2 tsp ground cumin
- 2 cups brown rice
- Sea salt and black pepper, to taste
- 1/2 tsp ground turmeric
- 2 tbsp fresh cilantro, finely chopped

Directions:
- Heat the sesame oil in a saucepan over medium-high heat.
- Once hot, cook the onion, peppers, parsnip, carrot and broccoli for about 3 minutes until aromatic.
- Add in the garlic and ground cumin; continue to cook for 30 seconds more until aromatic.
- Place the brown rice in a saucepan and cover with cold water by 2 inches. Bring to a boil. Turn the heat to a simmer and continue to cook for about 30 minutes or until tender.
- Stir the rice into the vegetable mixture; season with salt, black pepper and ground turmeric; garnish with fresh cilantro and serve immediately. Enjoy

181) EASY AMARANT GRITS WITH WALNUTS

Preparation Time: 35 minutes

Servings: 4

Ingredients:
- 2 cups water
- 2 cups coconut milk
- 1 cup amaranth
- 1 cinnamon stick
- 1 vanilla bean
- 4 tbsp maple syrup
- 4 tbsp walnuts, chopped

Directions:
- Bring the water and coconut milk to a boil over medium-high heat; add in the amaranth, cinnamon and vanilla and turn the heat to a simmer.
- Let it cook for about 30 minutes, stirring periodically to prevent the amaranth from sticking to the bottom of the pan.
- Top with maple syrup and walnuts. Enjoy

182) DELICIOUS BARLEY PILAF WITH WILD MUSHROOMS

Preparation Time: 45 minutes

Servings: 4

Ingredients:
- 2 tbsp vegan butter
- 1 small onion, chopped
- 1 tsp garlic, minced
- 1 jalapeno pepper, seeded and minced
- 1 pound wild mushrooms, sliced
- 1 cup medium pearl barley, rinsed
- 2 ¾ cups vegetable broth

Directions:
- Melt the vegan butter in a saucepan over medium-high heat.
- Once hot, cook the onion for about 3 minutes until just tender.
- Add in the garlic, jalapeno pepper, mushrooms; continue to sauté for 2 minutes or until aromatic.
- Add in the barley and broth, cover and continue to simmer for about 30 minutes. Once all the liquid has absorbed, allow the barley to rest for about 10 minutes fluff with a fork.
- Taste and adjust the seasonings. Enjoy

183) TASTY SWEET CORNBREAD MUFFINS

Preparation Time: 30 minutes — **Servings:** 8

Ingredients:
- 1 cup all-purpose flour
- 1 cup yellow cornmeal
- 1 tsp baking powder
- 1 tsp baking soda
- 1 tsp kosher salt
- 1/2 cup sugar
- 1/2 tsp ground cinnamon
- 1 1/2 cups almond milk
- 1/2 cup vegan butter, melted
- 2 tbsp applesauce

Directions:
- Start by preheating your oven to 420 degrees F. Now, spritz a muffin tin with a nonstick cooking spray.
- In a mixing bowl, thoroughly combine the flour, cornmeal, baking soda, baking powder, salt, sugar and cinnamon.
- Gradually add in the milk, butter and applesauce, whisking constantly to avoid lumps.
- Scrape the batter into the prepared muffin tin. Bake your muffins for about 25 minutes or until a tester inserted in the middle comes out dry and clean.
- Transfer them to a wire rack to rest for 5 minutes before unmolding and serving. Enjoy

184) ITALIAN ACRYLIC RICE PUDDING WITH DRIED FIGS

Preparation Time: 45 minutes — **Servings:** 4

Ingredients:
- 2 cups water
- 1 cup medium-grain white rice
- 3 ½ cups coconut milk
- 1/2 cup coconut sugar
- 1 cinnamon stick
- 1 vanilla bean
- 1/2 cup dried figs, chopped
- 4 tbsp coconut, shredded

Directions:
- In a saucepan, bring the water to a boil over medium-high heat. Immediately turn the heat to a simmer, add in the rice and let it cook for about 20 minutes.
- Add in the milk, sugar and spices and continue to cook for 20 minutes more, stirring constantly to prevent the rice from sticking to the pan.
- Top with dried figs and coconut; serve your pudding warm or at room temperature. Enjoy

185) SIMPLE POTAGE AU QUINOA

Preparation Time: 25 minutes — **Servings:** 4

Ingredients:
- 2 tbsp olive oil
- 1 onion, chopped
- 4 medium potatoes, peeled and diced
- 1 carrot, trimmed and diced
- 1 parsnip, trimmed and diced
- 1 jalapeno pepper, seeded and chopped
- 4 cups vegetable broth
- 1 cup quinoa
- Sea salt and ground white pepper, to taste

Directions:
- In a heavy-bottomed pot, heat the olive oil over medium-high heat. Sauté the onion, potatoes, carrots, parsnip and pepper for about 5 minutes or until they've softened.
- Add in the vegetable broth and quinoa; bring to a boil.
- Immediately turn the heat to a simmer for about 15 minutes or until the quinoa is tender.
- Season with salt and pepper to taste. Puree your potage with an immersion blender. Reheat the potage just before serving and enjoy

186) EASY SORGHUM BOWL WITH ALMONDS

Preparation Time: :15 minutes — **Servings:** 4

Ingredients:
- 1 cup sorghum
- 3 cups almond milk
- A pinch of sea salt
- A pinch of grated nutmeg
- 1/2 tsp ground cinnamon
- 1/4 tsp ground cardamom
- 1 tsp crystallized ginger
- 4 tbsp brown sugar
- 4 tbsp almonds, slivered

Directions:
- Place the sorghum, almond milk, salt, nutmeg, cinnamon, cardamom and crystallized ginger in a saucepan; simmer gently for about 15 minutes.
- Add in the brown sugar, stir and spoon the porridge into serving bowls.
- Top with almonds and serve immediately. Enjoy

Chapter 3. DINNER

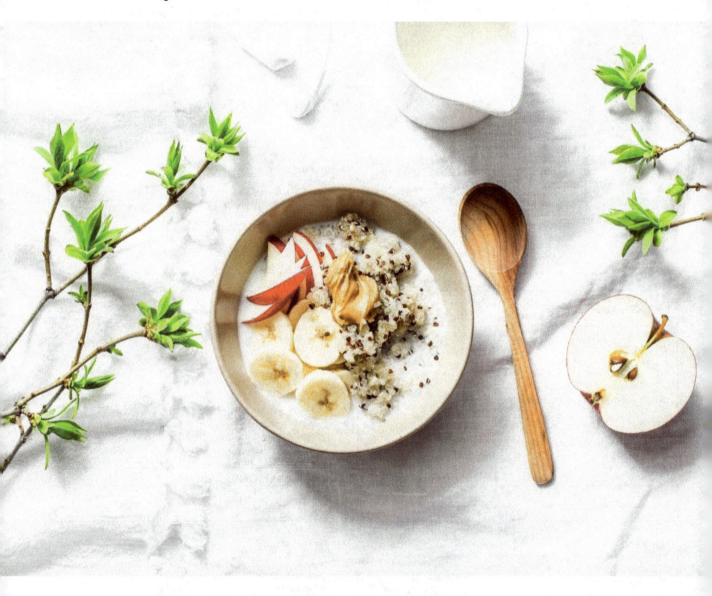

187) SIMPLE CAULIFLOWER RICE

Preparation Time: 10 minutes | **Servings:** 5

Ingredients:
- 2 medium heads cauliflower, stems and leaves removed
- 4 tbsp extra-virgin olive oil
- 4 garlic cloves, pressed
- 1/2 tsp red pepper flakes, crushed
- Sea salt and ground black pepper, to taste
- 1/4 cup flat-leaf parsley, roughly chopped

Directions:
- Pulse the cauliflower in a food processor with the S-blade until they're broken into "rice".
- Heat the olive oil in a saucepan over medium-high heat. Once hot, cook the garlic until fragrant or about 1 minute.
- Add in the cauliflower rice, red pepper, salt and black pepper and continue sautéing for a further 7 to 8 minutes.
- Taste, adjust the seasonings and garnish with fresh parsley. Enjoy

188) SIMPLE GARLICKY KALE

Preparation Time: 10 minutes | **Servings:** 4

Ingredients:
- 4 tbsp olive oil
- 4 cloves garlic, chopped
- 1 ½ pounds fresh kale, tough stems and ribs removed, torn into pieces
- 1 cup vegetable broth
- 1/2 tsp cumin seeds
- 1/2 tsp dried oregano
- 1/2 tsp paprika
- 1 tsp onion powder
- Sea salt and ground black pepper, to taste

Directions:
- In a saucepan, heat the olive oil over a moderately high heat. Now, sauté the garlic for about 1 minute or until aromatic.
- Add in the kale in batches, gradually adding the vegetable broth; stir to promote even cooking.
- Turn the heat to a simmer, add in the spices and let it cook for 5 to 6 minutes, until the kale leaves wilt.
- Serve warm and enjoy

189) ITALIAN ARTICHOKES BRAISED IN LEMON AND OLIVE OIL

Preparation Time: 35 minutes | **Servings:** 4

Ingredients:
- 1 ½ cups water
- 2 lemons, freshly squeezed
- 2 pounds artichokes, trimmed, tough outer leaves and chokes removed
- 1 handful fresh Italian parsley
- 2 thyme sprigs
- 2 rosemary sprigs
- 2 bay leaves
- 2 garlic cloves, chopped
- 1/3 cup olive oil
- Sea salt and ground black pepper, to taste
- 1/2 tsp red pepper flakes

Directions:
- Fill a bowl with water and add in the lemon juice. Place the cleaned artichokes in the bowl, keeping them completely submerged.
- In another small bowl, thoroughly combine the herbs and garlic. Rub your artichokes with the herb mixture.
- Pour the lemon water and olive oil in a saucepan; add the artichokes to the saucepan. Turn the heat to a simmer and continue to cook, covered, for about 30 minutes until the artichokes are crisp-tender.
- To serve, drizzle the artichokes with cooking juices, season them with the salt, black pepper and red pepper flakes. Enjoy

190) MEDITERRANEAN ROSEMARY AND GARLIC ROASTED CARROTS

Preparation Time: 25 minutes | **Servings:** 4

Ingredients:
- 2 pounds carrots, trimmed and halved lengthwise
- 4 tbsp olive oil
- 2 tbsp champagne vinegar
- 4 cloves garlic, minced
- 2 sprigs rosemary, chopped
- Sea salt and ground black pepper, to taste
- 4 tbsp pine nuts, chopped

Directions:
- Begin by preheating your oven to 400 degrees F.
- Toss the carrots with the olive oil, vinegar, garlic, rosemary, salt and black pepper. Arrange them in a single layer on a parchment-lined roasting sheet.
- Roast the carrots in the preheated oven for about 20 minutes, until fork-tender.
- Garnish the carrots with the pine nuts and serve immediately. Enjoy

191) EASY MEDITERRANEAN-STYLE GREEN BEANS

Preparation Time: 20 minutes **Servings:** 4

Ingredients:
- 2 tbsp olive oil
- 1 red bell pepper, seeded and diced
- 1 ½ pounds green beans
- 4 garlic cloves, minced
- 1/2 tsp mustard seeds
- 1/2 tsp fennel seeds
- 1 tsp dried dill weed
- 2 tomatoes, pureed
- 1 cup cream of celery soup
- 1 tsp Italian herb mix
- 1 tsp cayenne pepper
- Salt and freshly ground black pepper

Directions:
- Heat the olive oil in a saucepan over medium flame. Once hot, fry the peppers and green beans for about 5 minutes, stirring periodically to promote even cooking.
- Add in the garlic, mustard seeds, fennel seeds and dill and continue sautéing an additional 1 minute or until fragrant.
- Add in the pureed tomatoes, cream of celery soup, Italian herb mix, cayenne pepper, salt and black pepper. Continue to simmer, covered, for about 9 minutes or until the green beans are tender.
- Taste, adjust the seasonings and serve warm. Enjoy

192) SIMPLE ROASTED GARDEN VEGETABLES

Preparation Time: 45 minutes **Servings:** 4

Ingredients:
- 1 pound butternut squash, peeled and cut into 1-inch pieces
- 4 sweet potatoes, peeled and cut into 1-inch pieces
- 1/2 cup carrots, peeled and cut into 1-inch pieces
- 2 medium onions, cut into wedges
- 4 tbsp olive oil
- 1 tsp granulated garlic
- 1 tsp paprika
- 1 tsp dried rosemary
- 1 tsp mustard seeds
- Kosher salt and freshly ground black pepper, to taste

Directions:
- Start by preheating your oven to 420 degrees F.
- Toss the vegetables with the olive oil and spices. Arrange them on a parchment-lined roasting pan.
- Roast for about 25 minutes. Stir the vegetables and continue to cook for 20 minutes more.
- Enjoy

193) QUICK ROASTED KOHLRABI

Preparation Time: 30 minutes **Servings:** 4

Ingredients:
- 1 pound kohlrabi bulbs, peeled and sliced
- 4 tbsp olive oil
- 1/2 tsp mustard seeds
- 1 tsp celery seeds
- 1 tsp dried marjoram
- 1 tsp granulated garlic, minced
- Sea salt and ground black pepper, to taste
- 2 tbsp nutritional yeast

Directions:
- Start by preheating your oven to 450 degrees F.
- Toss the kohlrabi with the olive oil and spices until well coated. Arrange the kohlrabi in a single layer on a parchment-lined roasting pan.
- Bake the kohlrabi in the preheated oven for about 15 minutes; stir them and continue to cook an additional 15 minutes.
- Sprinkle nutritional yeast over the warm kohlrabi and serve immediately. Enjoy

194) SPECIAL CAULIFLOWER WITH TAHINI SAUCE

Preparation Time: 10 minutes **Servings:** 4

Ingredients:
- 1 cup water
- 2 pounds cauliflower florets
- Sea salt and ground black pepper, to taste
- 3 tbsp soy sauce
- 5 tbsp tahini
- 2 cloves garlic, minced
- 2 tbsp lemon juice

Directions:
- In a large saucepan, bring the water to a boil; then, add in the cauliflower and cook for about 6 minutes or until fork-tender; drain, season with salt and pepper and reserve.
- In a mixing bowl, thoroughly combine the soy sauce, tahini, garlic and lemon juice. Spoon the sauce over the cauliflower florets and serve.
- Enjoy

195) ITALIAN-STYLE HERB CAULIFLOWER MASH

Preparation Time: 25 minutes **Servings:** 4

Ingredients:
- 1 ½ pounds cauliflower florets
- 4 tbsp vegan butter
- 4 cloves garlic, sliced
- Sea salt and ground black pepper, to taste
- 1/4 cup plain oat milk, unsweetened
- 2 tbsp fresh parsley, roughly chopped

Directions:
- Steam the cauliflower florets for about 20 minutes; set it aside to cool.
- In a saucepan, melt the vegan butter over a moderately high heat; now, sauté the garlic for about 1 minute or until aromatic.
- Add the cauliflower florets to your food processor followed by the sautéed garlic, salt, black pepper and oat milk. Puree until everything is well incorporated.
- Garnish with fresh parsley leaves and serve hot. Enjoy

196) BEST GARLIC AND HERB MUSHROOM SKILLET

Preparation Time: 10 minutes **Servings:** 4

Ingredients:
- 4 tbsp vegan butter
- 1 ½ pounds oyster mushrooms halved
- 3 cloves garlic, minced
- 1 tsp dried oregano
- 1 tsp dried rosemary
- 1 tsp dried parsley flakes
- 1 tsp dried marjoram
- 1/2 cup dry white wine
- Kosher salt and ground black pepper, to taste

Directions:
- In a sauté pan, heat the olive oil over a moderately high heat.
- Now, sauté the mushrooms for 3 minutes or until they release the liquid. Add in the garlic and continue to cook for 30 seconds more or until aromatic.
- Stir in the spices and continue sautéing an additional 6 minutes, until your mushrooms are lightly browned.
- Enjoy

197) SIMPLE PAN-FRIED ASPARAGUS

Preparation Time: 10 minutes **Servings:** 4

Ingredients:
- 4 tbsp vegan butter
- 1 ½ pounds asparagus spears, trimmed
- 1/2 tsp cumin seeds, ground
- 1/4 tsp bay leaf, ground
- Sea salt and ground black pepper, to taste
- 1 tsp fresh lime juice

Directions:
- Melt the vegan butter in a saucepan over medium-high heat.
- Sauté the asparagus for about 3 to 4 minutes, stirring periodically to promote even cooking.
- Add in the cumin seeds, bay leaf, salt and black pepper and continue to cook the asparagus for 2 minutes more until crisp-tender.
- Drizzle lime juice over the asparagus and serve warm. Enjoy

198) EASY GINGERY CARROT MASH

Preparation Time: 25 minutes **Servings:** 4

Ingredients:
- 2 pounds carrots, cut into rounds
- 2 tbsp olive oil
- 1 tsp ground cumin
- Salt ground black pepper, to taste
- 1/2 tsp cayenne pepper
- 1/2 tsp ginger, peeled and minced
- 1/2 cup whole milk

Directions:
- Begin by preheating your oven to 400 degrees F.
- Toss the carrots with the olive oil, cumin, salt, black pepper and cayenne pepper. Arrange them in a single layer on a parchment-lined roasting sheet.
- Roast the carrots in the preheated oven for about 20 minutes, until crisp-tender.
- Add the roasted carrots, ginger and milk to your food processor; puree the ingredients until everything is well blended.
- Enjoy

199) ONLY MEDITERRANEAN-STYLE ROASTED ARTICHOKES

Preparation Time: 50 minutes **Servings:** 4

Ingredients:
- 4 artichokes, trimmed, tough outer leaves and chokes removed, halved
- 2 lemons, freshly squeezed
- 4 tbsp extra-virgin olive oil
- 4 cloves garlic, chopped
- 1 tsp fresh rosemary
- 1 tsp fresh basil
- 1 tsp fresh parsley
- 1 tsp fresh oregano
- Flaky sea salt and ground black pepper, to taste
- 1 tsp red pepper flakes
- 1 tsp paprika

Directions:
- Start by preheating your oven to 395 degrees F. Rub the lemon juice all over the entire surface of your artichokes.
- In a small mixing bowl, thoroughly combine the garlic with herbs and spices
- Place the artichoke halves in a parchment-lined baking dish, cut-side-up. Brush the artichokes evenly with the olive oil. Fill the cavities with the garlic/herb mixture.
- Bake for about 20 minutes. Now, cover them with aluminum foil and bake for a further 30 minutes. Serve warm and enjoy

200) ASIAN THAI-STYLE BRAISED KALE

Preparation Time: 10 minutes **Servings:** 4

Ingredients:
- 1 cup water
- 1 ½ pounds kale, tough stems and ribs removed, torn into pieces
- 2 tbsp sesame oil
- 1 tsp fresh garlic, pressed
- 1 tsp ginger, peeled and minced
- 1 Thai chili, chopped
- 1/2 tsp turmeric powder
- 1/2 cup coconut milk
- Kosher salt and ground black pepper, to taste

Directions:
- In a large saucepan, bring the water to a rapid boil. Add in the kale and let it cook until bright, about 3 minutes. Drain, rinse and squeeze dry.
- Wipe the saucepan with paper towels and preheat the sesame oil over a moderate heat. Once hot, cook the garlic, ginger and chili for approximately 1 minute or so, until fragrant.
- Add in the kale and turmeric powder and continue to cook for a further 1 minute or until heated through.
- Gradually pour in the coconut milk, salt and black pepper; continue to simmer until the liquid has thickened. Taste, adjust the seasonings and serve hot. Enjoy

201) SPECIAL SILKY KOHLRABI PUREE

Preparation Time: 30 minutes **Servings:** 4

Ingredients:
- 1 ½ pounds kohlrabi, peeled and cut into pieces
- 4 tbsp vegan butter
- Sea salt and freshly ground black pepper, to taste
- 1/2 tsp cumin seeds
- 1/2 tsp coriander seeds
- 1/2 cup soy milk
- 1 tsp fresh dill
- 1 tsp fresh parsley

Directions:
- Cook the kohlrabi in boiling salted water until soft, about 30 minutes; drain.
- Puree the kohlrabi with the vegan butter, salt, black pepper, cumin seeds and coriander seeds.
- Puree the ingredients with an immersion blender, gradually adding the milk. Top with fresh dill and parsley. Enjoy

202) TASTY CREAMY SAUTÉED SPINACH

Preparation Time: 15 minutes **Servings:** 4

Ingredients:
- 2 tbsp vegan butter
- 1 onion, chopped
- 1 tsp garlic, minced
- 1 ½ cups vegetable broth
- 2 pounds spinach, torn into pieces
- Sea salt and ground black pepper, to taste
- 1/4 tsp dried dill
- 1/4 tsp mustard seeds
- 1/2 tsp celery seeds
- 1 tsp cayenne pepper
- 1/2 cup oat milk

Directions:
- In a saucepan, melt the vegan butter over medium-high heat.
- Then, sauté the onion for about 3 minutes or until tender and translucent. Then, sauté the garlic for about 1 minute until aromatic.
- Add in the broth and spinach and bring to a boil.
- Turn the heat to a simmer. Add in the spices and continue to cook for 5 minutes longer.
- Add in the milk and continue to cook for 5 minutes more. Enjoy

203) BEST TOFU SKEWERS WITH SALSA VERDE AND SQUASH MASH

Preparation Time: 20 minutes

Servings: 4

Ingredients:

- 7 tbsp fresh cilantro, finely chopped
- 4 tbsp fresh basil, finely chopped
- 2 garlic cloves
- Juice of ½ lemon
- 4 tbsp capers
- 2/3 cup olive oil
- 1 lb extra firm tofu, cubed
- ½ tbsp sugar-free BBQ sauce
- 1 tbsp melted plant butter
- 3 cups butternut squash, cubed
- ½ cup cold plant butter
- 2 oz grated plant-based Parmesan

Directions:

- In a blender, add cilantro, basil, garlic, lemon juice, capers, olive oil, salt, and pepper. Process until smooth; set aside. Thread the tofu cubes on wooden skewers. Season with salt and brush with BBQ sauce. Melt plant butter in a grill pan and fry the tofu until browned. Remove to a plate. Pour the squash into a pot, add some lightly salted water, and bring the vegetable to a boil until soft, about 6 minutes. Drain and pour into a bowl. Add the cold plant butter, plant-based Parmesan cheese, salt, and black pepper. Mash the vegetable with an immersion blender until the consistency of mashed potatoes is achieved. Serve the tofu skewers with the mashed cauliflower and salsa verde

204) SPECIAL MUSHROOM LETTUCE WRAPS

Preparation Time: 25 minutes

Servings: 4

Ingredients:

- 2 tbsp plant butter
- 4 oz baby Bella mushrooms, sliced
- 1 ½ lb tofu, crumbled
- 1 iceberg lettuce, leaves extracted
- 1 cup grated plant-based cheddar
- 1 large tomato, sliced

Directions:

- Melt the plant butter in a skillet, add in mushrooms and sauté until browned and tender, about 6 minutes. Transfer to a plate. Add the tofu to the skillet and cook until brown, about 10 minutes. Spoon the tofu and mushrooms into the lettuce leaves, sprinkle with the plant-based cheddar cheese, and share the tomato slices on top. Serve the burger immediately

205) ORIGINAL GARLICKY RICE

Preparation Time: 20 minutes

Servings: 4

Ingredients:

- 4 tbsp olive oil
- 4 cloves garlic, chopped
- 1 ½ cups white rice
- 2 ½ cups vegetable broth

Directions:

- In a saucepan, heat the olive oil over a moderately high flame. Add in the garlic and sauté for about 1 minute or until aromatic.
- Add in the rice and broth. Bring to a boil; immediately turn the heat to a gentle simmer.
- Cook for about 15 minutes or until all the liquid has absorbed. Fluff the rice with a fork, season with salt and pepper and serve hot

206) CLASSIC BROWN RICE WITH VEGETABLES AND TOFU

Preparation Time: 45 minutes

Servings: 4

Ingredients:

- 4 tsp sesame seeds
- 2 spring garlic stalks, minced
- 1 cup spring onions, chopped
- 1 carrot, trimmed and sliced
- 1 celery rib, sliced
- 1/4 cup dry white wine
- 10 ounces tofu, cubed
- 1 ½ cups long-grain brown rice, rinsed thoroughly
- 2 tbsp soy sauce
- 2 tbsp tahini
- 1 tbsp lemon juice

Directions:

- In a wok or large saucepan, heat 2 tsp of the sesame oil over medium-high heat. Now, cook the garlic, onion, carrot and celery for about 3 minutes, stirring periodically to ensure even cooking.
- Add the wine to deglaze the pan and push the vegetables to one side of the wok. Add in the remaining sesame oil and fry the tofu for 8 minutes, stirring occasionally.
- Bring 2 ½ cups of water to a boil over medium-high heat. Bring to a simmer and cook the rice for about 30 minutes or until it is tender; fluff the rice and stir it with the soy sauce and tahini.
- Stir the vegetables and tofu into the hot rice; add a few drizzles of the fresh lemon juice and serve warm. Enjoy

207) SIMPLE AMARANTH PORRIDGE

Preparation Time: 35 minutes | **Servings:** 4

Ingredients:
- 3 cups water
- 1 cup amaranth
- 1/2 cup coconut milk
- 4 tbsp agave syrup
- A pinch of kosher salt
- A pinch of grated nutmeg

Directions:
- Bring the water to a boil over medium-high heat; add in the amaranth and turn the heat to a simmer.
- Let it cook for about 30 minutes, stirring periodically to prevent the amaranth from sticking to the bottom of the pan.
- Stir in the remaining ingredients and continue to cook for 1 to 2 minutes more until cooked through. Enjoy

208) CLASSIC COUNTRY CORNBREAD WITH SPINACH

Preparation Time: 50 minutes | **Servings:** 8

Ingredients:
- 1 tbsp flaxseed meal
- 1 cup all-purpose flour
- 1 cup yellow cornmeal
- 1/2 tsp baking soda
- 1/2 tsp baking powder
- 1 tsp kosher salt
- 1 tsp brown sugar
- A pinch of grated nutmeg
- 1 ¼ cups oat milk, unsweetened
- 1 tsp white vinegar
- 1/2 cup olive oil
- 2 cups spinach, torn into pieces

Directions:
- Start by preheating your oven to 420 degrees F. Now, spritz a baking pan with a nonstick cooking spray.
- To make the flax eggs, mix flaxseed meal with 3 tbsp of the water. Stir and let it sit for about 15 minutes.
- In a mixing bowl, thoroughly combine the flour, cornmeal, baking soda, baking powder, salt, sugar and grated nutmeg.
- Gradually add in the flax egg, oat milk, vinegar and olive oil, whisking constantly to avoid lumps. Afterwards, fold in the spinach.
- Scrape the batter into the prepared baking pan. Bake your cornbread for about 25 minutes or until a tester inserted in the middle comes out dry and clean.
- Let it stand for about 10 minutes before slicing and serving. Enjoy

209) SIMPLE RICE PUDDING WITH CURRANTS

Preparation Time: 45 minutes | **Servings:** 4

Ingredients:
- 1 ½ cups water
- 1 cup white rice
- 2 ½ cups oat milk, divided
- 1/2 cup white sugar
- A pinch of salt
- A pinch of grated nutmeg
- 1 tsp ground cinnamon
- 1/2 tsp vanilla extract
- 1/2 cup dried currants

Directions:
- In a saucepan, bring the water to a boil over medium-high heat. Immediately turn the heat to a simmer, add in the rice and let it cook for about 20 minutes.
- Add in the milk, sugar and spices and continue to cook for 20 minutes more, stirring constantly to prevent the rice from sticking to the pan.
- Top with dried currants and serve at room temperature. Enjoy

210) EASY MILLET PORRIDGE WITH SULTANAS

Preparation Time: 25 minutes | **Servings:** 3

Ingredients:
- 1 cup water
- 1 cup coconut milk
- 1 cup millet, rinsed
- 1/4 tsp grated nutmeg
- 1/4 tsp ground cinnamon
- 1 tsp vanilla paste
- 1/4 tsp kosher salt
- 2 tbsp agave syrup
- 4 tbsp sultana raisins

Directions:
- Place the water, milk, millet, nutmeg, cinnamon, vanilla and salt in a saucepan; bring to a boil.
- Turn the heat to a simmer and let it cook for about 20 minutes; fluff the millet with a fork and spoon into individual bowls.
- Serve with agave syrup and sultanas. Enjoy

211) ENGLISH QUINOA PORRIDGE WITH DRIED FIGS

Preparation Time: 25 minutes **Servings:** 3

Ingredients:
- 1 cup white quinoa, rinsed
- 2 cups almond milk
- 4 tbsp brown sugar
- A pinch of salt
- 1/4 tsp grated nutmeg
- 1/2 tsp ground cinnamon
- 1/2 tsp vanilla extract
- 1/2 cup dried figs, chopped

Directions:
- Place the quinoa, almond milk, sugar, salt, nutmeg, cinnamon and vanilla extract in a saucepan.
- Bring it to a boil over medium-high heat. Turn the heat to a simmer and let it cook for about 20 minutes; fluff with a fork.
- Divide between three serving bowls and garnish with dried figs. Enjoy

212) EASY BREAD PUDDING WITH RAISINS

Preparation Time: 1 hour **Servings:** 4

Ingredients:
- 4 cups day-old bread, cubed
- 1 cup brown sugar
- 4 cups coconut milk
- 1/2 tsp vanilla extract
- 1 tsp ground cinnamon
- 2 tbsp rum
- 1/2 cup raisins

Directions:
- Start by preheating your oven to 360 degrees F. Lightly oil a casserole dish with a nonstick cooking spray.
- Place the cubed bread in the prepared casserole dish.
- In a mixing bowl, thoroughly combine the sugar, milk, vanilla, cinnamon, rum and raisins. Pour the custard evenly over the bread cubes.
- Let it soak for about 15 minutes.
- Bake in the preheated oven for about 45 minutes or until the top is golden and set. Enjoy

213) SIMPLE BULGUR WHEAT SALAD

Preparation Time: 25 minutes **Servings:** 4

Ingredients:
- 1 cup bulgur wheat
- 1 ½ cups vegetable broth
- 1 tsp sea salt
- 1 tsp fresh ginger, minced
- 4 tbsp olive oil
- 1 onion, chopped
- 8 ounces canned garbanzo beans, drained
- 2 large roasted peppers, sliced
- 2 tbsp fresh parsley, roughly chopped

Directions:
- In a deep saucepan, bring the bulgur wheat and vegetable broth to a simmer; let it cook, covered, for 12 to 13 minutes.
- Let it stand for about 10 minutes and fluff with a fork.
- Add the remaining ingredients to the cooked bulgur wheat; serve at room temperature or well-chilled. Enjoy

214) QUICK RYE PORRIDGE WITH BLUEBERRY TOPPING

Preparation Time: 15 minutes **Servings:** 3

Ingredients:
- 1 cup rye flakes
- 1 cup water
- 1 cup coconut milk
- 1 cup fresh blueberries
- 1 tbsp coconut oil
- 6 dates, pitted

Directions:
- Add the rye flakes, water and coconut milk to a deep saucepan; bring to a boil over medium-high. Turn the heat to a simmer and let it cook for 5 to 6 minutes.
- In a blender or food processor, puree the blueberries with the coconut oil and dates.
- Ladle into three bowls and garnish with the blueberry topping.
- Enjoy

215) EXOTIC COCONUT SORGHUM PORRIDGE

Preparation Time: 15 minutes

Servings: 2

Ingredients:
- 1/2 cup sorghum
- 1 cup water
- 1/2 cup coconut milk
- 1/4 tsp grated nutmeg
- 1/4 tsp ground cloves
- 1/2 tsp ground cinnamon
- Kosher salt, to taste
- 2 tbsp agave syrup
- 2 tbsp coconut flakes

Directions:
- Place the sorghum, water, milk, nutmeg, cloves, cinnamon and kosher salt in a saucepan; simmer gently for about 15 minutes.
- Spoon the porridge into serving bowls. Top with agave syrup and coconut flakes. Enjoy

216) MAMMA'S AROMATIC RICE

Preparation Time: 20 minutes

Servings: 4

Ingredients:
- 3 tbsp olive oil
- 1 tsp garlic, minced
- 1 tsp dried oregano
- 1 tsp dried rosemary
- 1 bay leaf
- 1 ½ cups white rice
- 2 ½ cups vegetable broth
- Sea salt and cayenne pepper, to taste

Directions:
- In a saucepan, heat the olive oil over a moderately high flame. Add in the garlic, oregano, rosemary and bay leaf; sauté for about 1 minute or until aromatic.
- Add in the rice and broth. Bring to a boil; immediately turn the heat to a gentle simmer.
- Cook for about 15 minutes or until all the liquid has absorbed. Fluff the rice with a fork, season with salt and pepper and serve immediately.
- Enjoy

217) EVERYSEASONS SAVORY GRITS

Preparation Time: 35 minutes

Servings: 4

Ingredients:
- 2 tbsp vegan butter
- 1 sweet onion, chopped
- 1 tsp garlic, minced
- 4 cups water
- 1 cup stone-ground grits
- Sea salt and cayenne pepper, to taste

Directions:
- In a saucepan, melt the vegan butter over medium-high heat. Once hot, cook the onion for about 3 minutes or until tender.
- Add in the garlic and continue to sauté for 30 seconds more or until aromatic; reserve.
- Bring the water to a boil over a moderately high heat. Stir in the grits, salt and pepper. Turn the heat to a simmer, cover and continue to cook, for about 30 minutes or until cooked through.
- Stir in the sautéed mixture and serve warm. Enjoy

218) ONLY GREEK-STYLE BARLEY SALAD

Preparation Time: 35 minutes

Servings: 4

Ingredients:
- 1 cup pearl barley
- 2 ¾ cups vegetable broth
- 2 tbsp apple cider vinegar
- 4 tbsp extra-virgin olive oil
- 2 bell peppers, seeded and diced
- 1 shallot, chopped
- 2 ounces sun-dried tomatoes in oil, chopped
- 1/2 green olives, pitted and sliced
- 2 tbsp fresh cilantro, roughly chopped

Directions:
- Bring the barley and broth to a boil over medium-high heat; now, turn the heat to a simmer.
- Continue to simmer for about 30 minutes until all the liquid has absorbed; fluff with a fork.
- Toss the barley with the vinegar, olive oil, peppers, shallots, sun-dried tomatoes and olives; toss to combine well.
- Garnish with fresh cilantro and serve at room temperature or well-chilled. Enjoy

219) SPECIAL SWEET MAIZE MEAL PORRIDGE

Preparation Time: 15 minutes   **Servings:** 2

- 2 cups water
- 1/2 cup maize meal
- 1/4 tsp ground allspice
- 1/4 tsp salt
- 2 tbsp brown sugar
- 2 tbsp almond butter

- In a saucepan, bring the water to a boil; then, gradually add in the maize meal and turn the heat to a simmer.
- Add in the ground allspice and salt. Let it cook for 10 minutes.
- Add in the brown sugar and almond butter and gently stir to combine. Enjoy

220) DELICIOUS DAD'S MILLET MUFFINS

Preparation Time: 20 minutes   **Servings:** 8

Ingredients:
- 2 cup whole-wheat flour
- 1/2 cup millet
- 2 tsp baking powder
- 1/2 tsp salt
- 1 cup coconut milk
- 1/2 cup coconut oil, melted
- 1/2 cup agave nectar
- 1/2 tsp ground cinnamon
- 1/4 tsp ground cloves
- A pinch of grated nutmeg
- 1/2 cup dried apricots, chopped

- Begin by preheating your oven to 400 degrees F. Lightly oil a muffin tin with a nonstick oil.
- In a mixing bowl, mix all dry ingredients. In a separate bowl, mix the wet ingredients. Stir the milk mixture into the flour mixture; mix just until evenly moist and do not overmix your batter.
- Fold in the apricots and scrape the batter into the prepared muffin cups.
- Bake the muffins in the preheated oven for about 15 minutes, or until a tester inserted in the center of your muffin comes out dry and clean.
- Let it stand for 10 minutes on a wire rack before unmolding and serving. Enjoy

221) SIMPLE GINGER BROWN RICE

Preparation Time: 30 minutes   **Servings:** 4

Ingredients:
- 1 ½ cups brown rice, rinsed
- 2 tbsp olive oil
- 1 tsp garlic, minced
- 1 (1-inch) piece ginger, peeled and minced
- 1/2 tsp cumin seeds
- Sea salt and ground black pepper, to taste

- Place the brown rice in a saucepan and cover with cold water by 2 inches. Bring to a boil.
- Turn the heat to a simmer and continue to cook for about 30 minutes or until tender.
- In a sauté pan, heat the olive oil over medium-high heat. Once hot, cook the garlic, ginger and cumin seeds until aromatic.
- Stir the garlic/ginger mixture into the hot rice; season with salt and pepper and serve immediately

222) EVERYDAY CHILI BEAN AND BROWN RICE TORTILLAS

Preparation Time: 50 minutes   **Servings:** 4

Ingredients:
- 1 cups brown rice
- Salt and black pepper to taste
- 1 tbsp olive oil
- 1 medium red onion, chopped
- 1 green bell pepper, diced
- 2 garlic cloves, minced
- 1 tbsp chili powder
- 1 tsp cumin powder
- 1/8 tsp red chili flakes
- 1 (15 oz) can black beans, rinsed
- 4 whole-wheat flour tortillas, warmed
- 1 cup salsa
- 1 cup coconut cream for topping
- 1 cup grated plant-based cheddar

- Add 2 cups of water and brown rice to a medium pot, season with some salt, and cook over medium heat until the water absorbs and the rice is tender, 15 to 20 minutes.
- Heat the olive oil in a medium skillet over medium heat and sauté the onion, bell pepper, and garlic until softened and fragrant, 3 minutes.
- Mix in the chili powder, cumin powder, red chili flakes, and season with salt and black pepper. Cook for 1 minute or until the food releases fragrance. Stir in the brown rice, black beans, and allow warming through, 3 minutes. Lay the tortillas on a clean, flat surface and divide the rice mixture in the center of each. Top with the salsa, coconut cream, and plant cheddar cheese. Fold the sides and ends of the tortillas over the filling to secure. Serve immediately

223) EASY CASHEW BUTTERED QUESADILLAS WITH LEAFY GREENS

Preparation Time: 30 minutes

Servings: 4

Ingredients:
- 3 tbsp flax seed powder
- ½ cup cashew cream cheese
- 1 ½ tsp psyllium husk powder
- 1 tbsp coconut flour
- ½ tsp salt
- 1 tbsp cashew butter
- 5 oz grated plant-based cheddar
- 1 oz leafy greens

- Preheat oven to 400 F.
- In a bowl, mix flax seed powder with ½ cup water and allow sitting to thicken for 5 minutes. Whisk cashew cream cheese into the vegan "flax egg" until the batter is smooth. In another bowl, combine psyllium husk powder, coconut flour, and salt. Add the flour mixture to the flax egg batter and fold in until incorporated. Allow sitting for a few minutes. Line a baking sheet with wax paper and pour in the mixture. Spread and bake for 5-7 minutes. Slice into 8 pieces. Set aside.
- For the filling, spoon a little cashew butter into a skillet and place a tortilla in the pan. Sprinkle with some plant-based cheddar cheese, leafy greens, and cover with another tortilla. Brown each side of the quesadilla for 1 minute or until the cheese melts. Transfer to a plate. Repeat assembling the quesadillas using the remaining cashew butter. Serve

224) EVERYDAY ASPARAGUS WITH CREAMY PUREE

Preparation Time: 15 minutes

Servings: 4

Ingredients:
- 4 tbsp flax seed powder
- 2 oz plant butter, melted
- 3 oz cashew cream cheese
- ½ cup coconut cream
- Powdered chili pepper to taste
- 1 tbsp olive oil
- ½ lb asparagus, hard stalks removed
- 3 oz plant butter
- Juice of ½ a lemon

- In a safe microwave bowl, mix the flax seed powder with ½ cup water and set aside to thicken for 5 minutes. Warm the vegan "flax egg" in the microwave for 1-2 minutes, then pour it into a blender. Add in plant butter, cashew cream cheese, coconut cream, salt, and chili pepper. Puree until smooth.
- Heat olive oil in a saucepan and roast the asparagus until lightly charred. Season with salt and black pepper and set aside. Melt plant butter in a frying pan until nutty and golden brown. Stir in lemon juice and pour the mixture into a sauce cup. Spoon the creamy blend into the center of four serving plates and use the back of the spoon to spread out lightly. Top with the asparagus and drizzle the lemon butter on top. Serve immediately

225) SIMPLE KALE MUSHROOM GALETTE

Preparation Time: 35 minutes

Servings: 4

Ingredients:
- 1 tbsp flax seed powder
- ½ cup grated plant-based mozzarella
- 1 tbsp plant butter
- ½ cup almond flour
- ¼ cup coconut flour
- ½ tsp onion powder
- 1 tsp baking powder
- 3 oz cashew cream cheese, softened
- 1 garlic clove, finely minced
- Salt and black pepper to taste
- 1 cup kale, chopped
- 2 oz cremini mushrooms, sliced
- 2 oz grated plant-based mozzarella
- 1 oz grated plant-based Parmesan
- Olive oil for brushing

- Preheat oven to 375 F. Line a baking sheet with parchment paper and grease with cooking spray.
- In a bowl, mix flax seed powder with 3 tbsp water and allow sitting to thicken for 5 minutes. Place a pot over low heat, add in plant-based mozzarella and plant butter, and melt both whiles stirring continuously; remove. Stir in almond and coconut flours, onion powder, baking powder, and ¼ tsp salt. Pour in the vegan "flax egg" and combine until a quite sticky dough forms. Transfer dough to the baking sheet and cover with another parchment paper. Use a rolling pin to flatten into a 12-inch circle.
- After, remove the parchment paper and spread the cashew cream cheese on the dough, leaving about a 2-inch border around the edges. Sprinkle with garlic, salt, and black pepper. Spread kale on top of the cheese, followed by the mushrooms. Sprinkle the plant-based mozzarella and plant-based Parmesan cheese on top. Fold the ends of the crust over the filling and brush with olive oil. Bake until the cheese has melted and the crust golden brown, about 25-30 minutes. Slice and serve with arugula salad

226) GENOVESE FOCACCIA WITH MIXED MUSHROOMS

Preparation Time: 35 minutes

Servings: 4

Ingredients:
- 2 tbsp flax seed powder
- ½ cup tofu mayonnaise
- ¾ cup almond flour
- 1 tbsp psyllium husk powder
- 1 tsp baking powder
- 2 oz mixed mushrooms, sliced
- 1 tbsp plant-based basil pesto
- 2 tbsp olive oil
- Salt and black pepper to taste
- ½ cup coconut cream
- ¾ cup grated plant-based Parmesan

Directions:
- Preheat oven to 350 F.
- Combine flax seed powder with 6 tbsp water and allow sitting to thicken for 5 minutes. Whisk in tofu mayonnaise, almond flour, psyllium husk powder, baking powder, and salt. Allow sitting for 5 minutes. Pour the batter into a baking sheet and spread out with a spatula. Bake for 10 minutes.
- In a bowl, mix mushrooms with pesto, olive oil, salt, and black pepper. Remove the crust from the oven and spread the coconut cream on top. Add the mushroom mixture and plant-based Parmesan cheese. Bake the pizza further until the cheese has melted, 5-10 minutes. Slice and serve with salad

227) VEGETARIAN SEITAN CAKES WITH BROCCOLI MASH

Preparation Time: 30 minutes

Servings: 4

Ingredients:
- 1 tbsp flax seed powder
- 1 ½ lb crumbled seitan
- ½ white onion
- 2 oz olive oil
- 1 lb broccoli
- 5 oz cold plant butter
- 2 oz grated plant-based Parmesan
- 4 oz plant butter, room temperature
- 2 tbsp lemon juice

Directions:
- Preheat oven to 220 F. In a bowl, mix the flax seed powder with 3 tbsp water and allow sitting to thicken for 5 minutes. When the vegan "flax egg" is ready, add in crumbled seitan, white onion, salt, and pepper. Mix and mold out 6-8 cakes out of the mixture. Melt plant butter in a skillet and fry the patties on both sides until golden brown. Remove onto a wire rack to cool slightly.
- Pour salted water into a pot, bring to a boil, and add in broccoli. Cook until the broccoli is tender but not too soft. Drain and transfer to a bowl. Add in cold plant butter, plant-based Parmesan, salt, and pepper. Puree the ingredients until smooth and creamy. Set aside. Mix the soft plant butter with lemon juice, salt, and pepper in a bowl. Serve the seitan cakes with the broccoli mash and lemon butter

228) SPECIAL SPICY CHEESE WITH TOFU BALLS

Preparation Time: 40 minutes

Servings: 4

Ingredients:
- 1/3 cup tofu mayonnaise
- ¼ cup pickled jalapenos
- 1 tsp paprika powder
- 1 tbsp mustard powder
- 1 pinch cayenne pepper
- 4 oz grated plant-based cheddar
- 1 tbsp flax seed powder
- 2 ½ cup crumbled tofu
- 2 tbsp plant butter

Directions:
- In a bowl, mix tofu mayonnaise, jalapeños, paprika, mustard powder, cayenne powder, and plant-based cheddar cheese; set aside. In another bowl, combine flax seed powder with 3 tbsp water and allow absorbing for 5 minutes. Add the vegan "flax egg" to the cheese mixture, crumbled tofu, salt, and pepper and combine well. Form meatballs out of the mix. Melt plant butter in a skillet and fry the tofu balls until browned. Serve the tofu balls with roasted cauliflower mash

229) TASTY QUINOA AND VEGGIE BURGERS

Preparation Time: 35 minutes

Servings: 4

Ingredients:
- 1 cup quick-cooking quinoa
- 1 tbsp olive oil
- 1 shallot, chopped
- 2 tbsp chopped fresh celery
- 1 garlic clove, minced
- 1 (15 oz) can pinto beans, drained
- 2 tbsp whole-wheat flour
- ¼ cup chopped fresh basil
- 2 tbsp pure maple syrup
- 4 whole-grain hamburger buns, split
- 4 small lettuce leaves for topping
- ½ cup tofu mayonnaise for topping

Directions:
- Cook the quinoa with 2 cups of water in a medium pot until the liquid absorbs, 10 to 15 minutes. Heat the olive oil in a medium skillet over medium heat and sauté the shallot, celery, and garlic until softened and fragrant, 3 minutes.
- Transfer the quinoa and shallot mixture to a medium bowl and add the pinto beans, flour, basil, maple syrup, salt, and black pepper. Mash and mold 4 patties out of the mixture and set aside.
- Heat a grill pan to medium heat and lightly grease with cooking spray. Cook the patties on both sides until light brown, compacted, and cooked through, 10 minutes. Place the patties between the burger buns and top with the lettuce and tofu mayonnaise. Serve

230) EASY BAKED TOFU WITH ROASTED PEPPERS

Preparation Time: 20 minutes **Servings:** 4

Ingredients:
- 3 oz cashew cream cheese
- ¾ cup tofu mayonnaise
- 2 oz cucumber, diced
- 1 large tomato, chopped
- 2 tsp dried parsley
- 4 medium orange bell peppers
- 2 ½ cups cubed tofu
- 1 tbsp melted plant butter
- 1 tsp dried basil

Directions:
- Preheat the oven's broiler to 450 F and line a baking sheet with parchment paper. In a salad bowl, combine cashew cream cheese, tofu mayonnaise, cucumber, tomato, salt, pepper, and parsley. Refrigerate.
- Arrange the bell peppers and tofu on the baking sheet, drizzle with melted plant butter, and season with basil, salt, and pepper. Bake for 10-15 minutes or until the peppers have charred lightly and the tofu browned. Remove from the oven and serve with the salad

231) SIMPLE ZOODLE BOLOGNESE

Preparation Time: 45 minutes **Servings:** 4

Ingredients:
- 3 oz olive oil
- 1 white onion, chopped
- 1 garlic clove, minced
- 3 oz carrots, chopped
- 3 cups crumbled tofu
- 2 tbsp tomato paste
- 1 ½ cups crushed tomatoes
- Salt and black pepper to taste
- 1 tbsp dried basil
- 1 tbsp vegan Worcestershire sauce
- 2 lb zucchini, spiralized
- 2 tbsp plant butter

Directions:
- Pour olive oil into a saucepan and heat over medium heat. Add in onion, garlic, and carrots and sauté for 3 minutes or until the onions are soft and the carrots caramelized. Pour in tofu, tomato paste, tomatoes, salt, pepper, basil, and Worcestershire sauce. Stir and cook for 15 minutes. Mix in some water if the mixture is too thick and simmer further for 20 minutes. Melt plant butter in a skillet and toss in the zoodles quickly, about 1 minute. Season with salt and black pepper. Divide into serving plates and spoon the Bolognese on top. Serve immediately

232) SPECIAL ZUCCHINI BOATS WITH VEGAN CHEESE

Preparation Time: 40 minutes **Servings:** 2

Ingredients:
- 1 medium-sized zucchini
- 4 tbsp plant butter
- 2 garlic cloves, minced
- 1 ½ oz baby kale
- Salt and black pepper to taste
- 2 tbsp unsweetened tomato sauce
- 1 cup grated plant-based mozzarella
- Olive oil for drizzling

Directions:
- Preheat oven to 375 F.
- Use a knife to slice the zucchini in halves and scoop out the pulp with a spoon into a plate. Keep the flesh. Grease a baking sheet with cooking spray and place the zucchini boats on top. Put the plant butter in a skillet and melt over medium heat.
- Sauté the garlic for 1 minute. Add in kale and zucchini pulp. Cook until the kale wilts; season with salt and black pepper. Spoon tomato sauce into the boats and spread to coat the bottom evenly. Then, spoon the kale mixture into the zucchinis and sprinkle with the plant-based mozzarella cheese. Bake for 20-25 minutes. Serve immediately

233) SPECIAL ROASTED BUTTERNUT SQUASH WITH CHIMICHURRI

Preparation Time: 15 minutes **Servings:** 4

Ingredients:
- Zest and juice of 1 lemon
- ½ medium red bell pepper, chopped
- 1 jalapeno pepper, chopped
- 1 cup olive oil
- ½ cup chopped fresh parsley
- 2 garlic cloves, minced
- 1 lb butternut squash
- 1 tbsp plant butter, melted
- 3 tbsp toasted pine nuts

Directions:
- In a bowl, add the lemon zest and juice, red bell pepper, jalapeno, olive oil, parsley, garlic, salt, and black pepper. Use an immersion blender to grind the ingredients until your desired consistency is achieved; set aside the chimichurri.
- Slice the butternut squash into rounds and remove the seeds. Drizzle with the plant butter and season with salt and black pepper. Preheat a grill pan over medium heat and cook the squash for 2 minutes on each side or until browned. Remove the squash to serving plates, scatter the pine nuts on top, and serve with the chimichurri and red cabbage salad

Chapter 4. DESSERTS

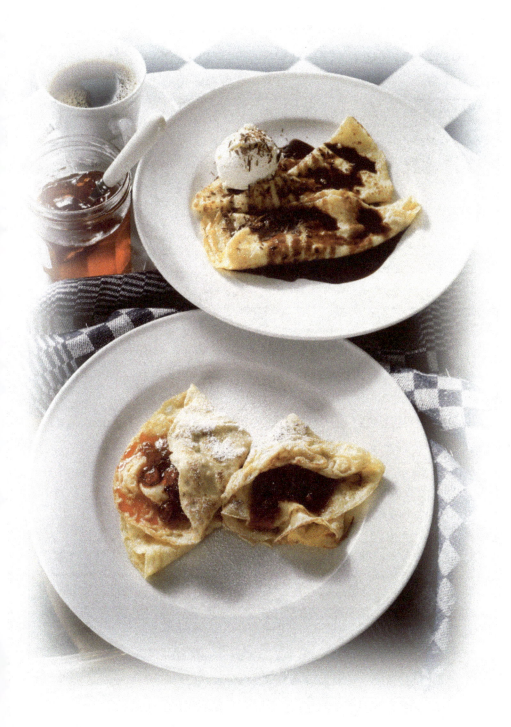

234) MILK CHOCOLATE FUDGE WITH NUTS

Preparation Time: 10 minutes + cooling time

Servings: 4

Ingredients:
- 3 cups chocolate chips
- ¼ cup thick coconut milk
- 1 ½ tsp vanilla extract
- A pinch salt
- 1 cup chopped mixed nuts

Directions:
- Line a square pan with baking paper. Melt the chocolate chips, coconut milk, and vanilla in a medium pot over low heat. Mix in the salt and nuts until well distributed and pour the mixture into the square pan. Refrigerate for at least 2 hours. Remove from the fridge, cut into squares, and serve

235) NOT TOO SWEET CHOCOLATE AND PEANUT BUTTER COOKIES

Preparation Time: 15 minutes + cooling time

Servings: 4

Ingredients:
- 1 tbsp flaxseed powder
- 1 cup pure date sugar + for dusting
- ½ cup vega butter, softened
- ½ cup creamy peanut butter
- 1 tsp vanilla extract
- 1 ¾ cup whole-wheat flour
- 1 tsp baking soda
- ¼ tsp salt
- ¼ cup unsweetened chocolate chips

Directions:
- In a small bowl, mix the flaxseed powder with 3 tbsp water and allow thickening for 5 minutes to make the vegan "flax egg." In a medium bowl, whisk the date sugar, plant butter, and peanut butter until light and fluffy. Mix in the flax egg and vanilla until combined. Add in flour, baking soda, salt, and whisk well again. Fold in chocolate chips, cover the bowl with plastic wrap, and refrigerate for 1 hour.
- Preheat oven to 375 F and line a baking sheet with parchment paper. Use a cookie sheet to scoop mounds of the batter onto the sheet with 1-inch intervals. Bake for 10 minutes. Remove the cookies from the oven, cool for 3 minutes, roll in some date sugar, and serve

236) SPECIAL MIXED BERRY YOGURT ICE POPS

Preparation Time: 5 minutes + chilling time

Servings: 6

Ingredients:
- 2/3 cup avocado, halved and pitted
- 2/3 cup frozen berries, thawed
- 1 cup dairy-free yogurt
- ½ cup coconut cream
- 1 tsp vanilla extract

Directions:
- Pour the avocado pulp, berries, dairy-free yogurt, coconut cream, and vanilla extract. Process until smooth. Pour into ice pop sleeves and freeze for 8 or more hours. Enjoy the ice pops when ready

237) EVERYDAY HOLIDAY PECAN TART

Preparation Time: 50 minutes + cooling time

Servings: 4

Ingredients:
- 4 tbsp flaxseed powder
- 1/3 cup whole-wheat flour
- ½ tsp salt
- ¼ cup cold plant butter, crumbled
- 3 tbsp pure malt syrup
- For the filling:
- 3 tbsp flaxseed powder + 9 tbsp water
- 2 cups toasted pecans, chopped
- 1 cup light corn syrup
- ½ cup pure date sugar
- 1 tbsp pure pomegranate molasses
- 4 tbsp plant butter, melted
- ½ tsp salt
- 2 tsp vanilla extract

Directions:
- Preheat oven to 350 F. In a bowl, mix the flaxseed powder with 12 tbsp water and allow thickening for 5 minutes. Do this for the filling's vegan "flax egg" too in a separate bowl. In a bowl, combine flour and salt. Add in plant butter and whisk until crumbly. Pour in the crust's vegan "flax egg" and maple syrup and mix until smooth dough forms. Flatten the dough on a flat surface, cover with plastic wrap, and refrigerate for 1 hour. Dust a working surface with flour, remove the dough onto the surface, and using a rolling pin, flatten the dough into a 1-inch diameter circle. Lay the dough on a greased pie pan and press to fit the shape of the pan. Trim the edges of the pan. Lay a parchment paper on the dough, pour on some baking beans and bake for 20 minutes. Remove, pour out baking beans, and allow cooling.
- In a bowl, mix the filling's vegan "flax egg," pecans, corn syrup, date sugar, pomegranate molasses, plant butter, salt, and vanilla. Pour and spread the mixture on the piecrust. Bake for 20 minutes or until the filling sets. Remove from the oven, decorate with more pecans, slice, and cool. Slice and serve

238) TROPICAL COCONUT CHOCOLATE BARKS

Preparation Time: 35 minutes

Servings: 4

- 1/3 cup coconut oil, melted
- ¼ cup almond butter, melted
- 2 tbsp unsweetened coconut flakes.
- 1 tsp pure maple syrup
- A pinch of ground rock salt
- ¼ cup unsweetened cocoa nibs

❖ Line a baking tray with baking paper and set aside. In a medium bowl, mix the coconut oil, almond butter, coconut flakes, maple syrup, and fold in the rock salt and cocoa nibs. Pour and spread the mixture on the baking sheet, chill in the refrigerator for 20 minutes or until firm. Remove the dessert, break into shards, and enjoy. Preserve extras in the refrigerator

239) EASY NUTTY DATE CAKE

Preparation Time: 1 hour 30 minutes

Servings: 4

- ½ cup cold plant butter, cut into pieces
- 1 tbsp flaxseed powder
- ½ cup whole-wheat flour
- ¼ cup chopped pecans and walnuts
- 1 tsp baking powder
- 1 tsp baking soda
- 1 tsp cinnamon powder
- 1 tsp salt
- 1/3 cup pitted dates, chopped
- ½ cup pure date sugar
- 1 tsp vanilla extract
- ¼ cup pure date syrup for drizzling.

❖ Preheat oven to 350 F and lightly grease a baking dish with some plant butter. In a small bowl, mix the flaxseed powder with 3 tbsp water and allow thickening for 5 minutes to make the vegan "flax egg."

❖ In a food processor, add the flour, nuts, baking powder, baking soda, cinnamon powder, and salt. Blend until well combined. Add 1/3 cup of water, dates, date sugar, and vanilla. Process until smooth with tiny pieces of dates evident.

❖ Pour the batter into the baking dish and bake in the oven for 1 hour and 10 minutes or until a toothpick inserted comes out clean. Remove the dish from the oven, invert the cake onto a serving platter to cool, drizzle with the date syrup, slice, and serve

240) DELICIOUS BERRY CUPCAKES WITH CASHEW CHEESE ICING

Preparation Time: 35 minutes + cooling time

Servings: 4

- 2 cups whole-wheat flour
- ¼ cup corn-starch
- 2 ½ tsp baking powder
- 1 ½ cups pure date sugar
- ½ tsp salt
- ¾ cup plant butter, softened
- 3 tsp vanilla extract
- 1 cup strawberries, pureed
- 1 cup oat milk, room temperature
- ¾ cup cashew cream
- 2 tbsp coconut oil, melted
- 3 tbsp pure maple syrup
- 1 tsp vanilla extract
- 1 tsp freshly squeezed lemon juice

❖ Preheat the oven to 350 F and line a 12-holed muffin tray with cupcake liners. Set aside.

❖ In a bowl, mix flour, corn-starch, baking powder, date sugar, and salt. Whisk in plant butter, vanilla extract, strawberries, and oat milk until well combined. Divide the mixture into the muffin cups two-thirds way up and bake for 20-25 minutes. Allow cooling while you make the frosting.

❖ In a blender, add cashew cream, coconut oil, maple syrup, vanilla, and lemon juice. Process until smooth. Pour the frosting into a medium bowl and chill for 30 minutes. Transfer the mixture into a piping bag and swirl mounds of the frosting onto the cupcakes. Serve immediately

241) EXOTIC COCONUT AND CHOCOLATE CAKE

Preparation Time: 40 minutes + cooling time

Servings: 4

Ingredients:

- 2/3 cup toasted almond flour
- ¼ cup unsalted plant butter, melted
- 2 cups chocolate bars, cubed
- 2 ½ cups coconut cream
- Fresh berries for topping

❖ Lightly grease a 9-inch springform pan with some plant butter and set aside.

❖ Mix the almond flour and plant butter in a medium bowl and pour the mixture into the springform pan. Use the spoon to spread and press the mixture into the bottom of the pan. Place in the refrigerator to firm for 30 minutes.

❖ Meanwhile, pour the chocolate in a safe microwave bowl and melt for 1 minute stirring every 30 seconds. Remove from the microwave and mix in the coconut cream and maple syrup.

❖ Remove the cake pan from the oven, pour the chocolate mixture on top, and shake the pan and even the layer. Chill further for 4 to 6 hours. Take out the pan from the fridge, release the cake and garnish with the raspberries or strawberries. Slice and serve

242) ITALIAN BERRY MACEDONIA WITH MINT

Preparation Time: 20 minutes

Servings: 4

Ingredients:
- ¼ cup lemon juice
- 4 tsp agave syrup
- 2 cups chopped pears
- 2 cups chopped strawberries
- 3 cups mixed berries
- 8 fresh mint leaves

Directions:
- Chop half of the mint leaves; reserve.
- In a large bowl, combine together pears, strawberries, raspberries, blackberries, and half of the mint leaves. Divide the Macedonia salad between 4 small cups. Top with lemon juice, agave syrup, and mint leaves and serve chilled

243) SPECIAL CINNAMON PUMPKIN PIE

Preparation Time: 1 hr 10 min + cooling time

Servings: 4

Ingredients:
- For the piecrust:
- 4 tbsp flaxseed powder
- 1/3 cup whole-wheat flour
- ½ tsp salt
- ¼ cup cold plant butter, crumbled
- 3 tbsp pure malt syrup
- For the filling:
- 2 tbsp flaxseed powder + 6 tbsp water
- 4 tbsp plant butter
- ¼ cup pure maple syrup
- ¼ cup pure date sugar
- 1 tsp cinnamon powder
- ½ tsp ginger powder
- 1/8 tsp cloves powder
- 1 (15 oz) can pumpkin purée
- 1 cup almond milk

Directions:
- Preheat oven to 350 F. In a bowl, mix flaxseed powder with 12 tbsp water and allow thickening for 5 minutes. Do this for the filling's vegan "flax egg" too in another bowl. In a bowl, combine flour and salt. Add in plant butter and whisk until crumbly. Pour in crust's vegan "flax egg," maple syrup, vanilla, and mix until smooth dough forms. Flatten, cover with plastic wrap, and refrigerate for 1 hour.
- Dust a working surface with flour, remove the dough onto the surface and flatten it into a 1-inch diameter circle. Lay the dough on a greased pie pan and press to fit the shape of the pan. Use a knife to trim the edges of the pan. Lay a parchment paper on the dough, pour on some baking beans and bake for 15-20 minutes. Remove, pour out the baking beans, and allow cooling. In a bowl, whisk filling's flaxseed, butter, maple syrup, date sugar, cinnamon powder, ginger powder, cloves powder, pumpkin puree, and almond milk. Pour the mixture onto the piecrust and bake for 35-40 minutes

244) EVERYTIME PARTY MATCHA AND HAZELNUT CHEESECAKE

Preparation Time: 20 minutes + cooling time

Servings: 4

Ingredients:
- 2/3 cup toasted rolled oats
- ¼ cup plant butter, melted
- 3 tbsp pure date sugar
- 6 oz cashew cream cheese
- ¼ cup almond milk
- 1 tbsp matcha powder
- ¼ cup just-boiled water
- 3 tsp agar agar powder
- 2 tbsp toasted hazelnuts, chopped

Directions:
- Process the oats, butter, and date sugar in a blender until smooth.
- Pour the mixture into a greased 9-inch springform pan and press the mixture onto the bottom of the pan. Refrigerate for 30 minutes until firm while you make the filling.
- In a large bowl, using an electric mixer, whisk the cashew cream cheese until smooth. Beat in the almond milk and mix in the matcha powder until smooth.
- Mix the boiled water and agar agar until dissolved and whisk this mixture into the creamy mix. Fold in the hazelnuts until well distributed. Remove the cake pan from the fridge and pour in the cream mixture. Shake the pan to ensure a smooth layering on top. Refrigerate further for at least 3 hours. Take out the cake pan, release the cake, slice, and serve

245) ITALIAN PISTACHIOS AND CHOCOLATE POPSICLES

Preparation Time: 5 minutes + cooling time

Servings: 4

Ingredients:
- ½ cup chocolate chips, melted
- 1 ½ cups oat milk
- 1 tbsp unsweetened cocoa powder
- 3 tbsp pure date syrup
- 1 tsp vanilla extract
- A handful of pistachios, chopped

Directions:
- In a blender, add chocolate, oat milk, cocoa powder, date syrup, vanilla, pistachios, and process until smooth. Divide the mixture into popsicle molds and freeze for 3 hours. Dip the popsicle molds in warm water to loosen the popsicles and pull out the popsicles

246) ENGLISH OATMEAL COOKIES WITH HAZELNUTS

Preparation Time: 15 minutes

Servings: 2

Ingredients:
- 1 ½ cups whole-grain flour
- 1 tsp baking powder
- ⅛ tsp salt
- 1 tsp ground cinnamon
- ¼ tsp ground nutmeg
- 1 ½ cups old-fashioned oats
- 1 cup chopped hazelnuts
- ½ cup plant butter, melted
- ½ cup pure maple syrup
- ¼ cup pure date sugar
- 2 tsp pure vanilla extract

Directions:
- Preheat oven to 360 F.
- Combine the flour, baking powder, salt, cinnamon, and nutmeg in a bowl. Add in oats and hazelnuts. In another bowl, whisk the butter, maple syrup, sugar, and vanilla. Pour over the flour mixture. Mix well. Spoon a small ball of cookie dough on a baking sheet and press down with a fork. Bake for 10-12 minutes, until browned. Let completely cool on a rack

247) TROPICAL COCONUT CHOCOLATE TRUFFLES

Preparation Time: 1 hour 15 minutes

Servings: 12

Ingredients:
- 1 cup raw cashews, soaked overnight
- ¾ cup pitted cherries
- 2 tbsp coconut oil
- 1 cup shredded coconut
- 2 tbsp cocoa powder

Directions:
- Line a baking sheet with parchment paper and set aside.
- Blend cashews, cherries, coconut oil, half of the shredded coconut, and cocoa powder in a food processor until ingredients are evenly mixed. Spread the remaining shredded coconut on a dish. Mold the mixture into 12 truffle shapes. Roll the truffles in the coconut dish, shaking off any excess, then arrange on the prepared baking sheet. Refrigerate for 1 hour

248) DELICIOUS LAYERED RASPBERRY AND TOFU CUPS

Preparation Time: 60 minutes

Servings: 4

Ingredients:
- ½ cup unsalted raw cashews
- 3 tbsp pure date sugar
- ½ cup soy milk
- ¾ cup firm silken tofu, drained
- 1 tsp vanilla extract
- 2 cups sliced raspberries
- 1 tsp fresh lemon juice
- Fresh mint leaves

Directions:
- Grind the cashews and 3 tbsp of date sugar in a blender until a fine powder is obtained. Pour in soy milk and blitz until smooth. Add in tofu and vanilla and pulse until creamy. Remove to a bowl and refrigerate covered for 30 minutes.
- In a bowl, mix the raspberries, lemon juice, and remaining date sugar. Let sit for 20 minutes. Assemble by alternating into small cups, one layer of raspberries and one layer of cashew cream, ending with the cashew cream. Serve garnished with mint leaves

249) EASY CASHEW AND CRANBERRY TRUFFLES

Preparation Time: 15 minutes **Servings:** 4

Ingredients:
- 2 cups fresh cranberries
- 2 tbsp pure date syrup
- 1 tsp vanilla extract
- 16 oz cashew cream
- 4 tbsp plant butter
- 3 tbsp unsweetened cocoa powder
- 2 tbsp pure date sugar

Directions:
- Set a silicone egg tray aside. Puree the cranberries, date syrup, and vanilla in a blender until smooth.
- Add the cashew cream and plant butter to a medium pot. Heat over medium heat until the mixture is well combined. Turn the heat off. Mix in the cranberry mixture and divide the mixture into the muffin holes. Refrigerate for 40 minutes or until firm. Remove the tray and pop out the truffles.
- Meanwhile, mix the cocoa powder and date sugar on a plate. Roll the truffles in the mixture until well dusted and serve

250) COCONUT PEACH TART

Preparation Time: 10 minutes **Servings:** 8

Ingredients:
- ½ cup rolled oats
- 1 cup cashews
- 1 cup soft pitted dates
- 1 cup canned coconut milk
- 2 large peaches, chopped
- ½ cup shredded coconut

Directions:
- In a food processor, pulse the oats, cashews, and dates until a dough-like mixture forms. Press down into a greased baking pan.
- Pulse the coconut milk, ½ cup water, peaches, and shredded coconut in the food processor until smooth. Pour this mixture over the crust and spread evenly. Freeze for 30 minutes. Soften 15 minutes before serving. Top with whipped coconut cream and shredded coconut

251) TROPICAL MANGO MUFFINS WITH CHOCOLATE CHIPS

Preparation Time: 40 minutes **Servings:** 12

Ingredients:
- Ingredients for 12 servings
- 2 medium mangoes, chopped
- 1 cup non-dairy milk
- 2 tbsp almond butter
- 1 tsp apple cider vinegar
- 1 tsp pure vanilla extract
- 1 ¼ cups whole-wheat flour
- ½ cup rolled oats
- ¼ cup coconut sugar
- 1 tsp baking powder
- ½ tsp baking soda
- ½ cup unsweetened cocoa powder
- ¼ cup sesame seeds
- A pinch of salt
- ¼ cup dark chocolate chips

Directions:
- Preheat oven to 360 F.
- In a food processor, put the mangoes, milk, almond butter, vinegar, and vanilla. Blend until smooth.
- In a bowl, combine the flour, oats, sugar, baking powder, baking soda, cocoa powder, sesame seeds, salt, and chocolate chips. Pour into the mango mixture and mix. Scoop into greased muffin cups and bake for 20-25 minutes. Let cool completely before removing from the cups

252) EASY MAPLE RICE PUDDING

Preparation Time: 30 minutes **Servings:** 4

Ingredients:
- 1 cup short-grain brown rice
- 1 ¾ cups non-dairy milk
- 4 tbsp pure maple syrup
- 1 tsp vanilla extract
- A pinch of salt
- ¼ cup dates, pitted and chopped

Directions:
- In a pot over medium heat, place the rice, milk, 1 ½ cups water, maple, vanilla, and salt. Bring to a boil, then reduce the heat. Cook for 20 minutes, stirring occasionally. Mix in dates and cook for another 5 minutes. Serve chilled in cups

253) DELICIOUS VANILLA COOKIES WITH POPPY SEEDS

Preparation Time: 15 minutes

Servings: 3

Ingredients:
- ¾ cup plant butter, softened
- ½ cup pure date sugar
- 1 tsp pure vanilla extract
- 2 tbsp pure maple syrup
- 2 cups whole-grain flour
- ¾ cup poppy seeds, lightly toasted

Directions:
- Beat the butter and sugar in a bowl until creamy and fluffy. Add in vanilla, and maple syrup, blend. Stir in flour and poppy seeds. Wrap the dough in a cylinder and cover it with plastic foil. Let chill in the fridge.
- Preheat oven to 330 F. Cut the dough into thin circles and arrange on a baking sheet. Bake for 12 minutes, until light brown. Let completely cool before serving

254) BEST KIWI AND PEANUT BARS

Preparation Time: 5 minutes

Servings: 9

Ingredients:
- 2 kiwis, mashed
- 1 tbsp maple syrup
- ½ tsp vanilla extract
- 2 cups old-fashioned rolled oats
- ½ tsp salt
- ¼ cup chopped peanuts

Directions:
- Preheat oven to 360 F.
- In a bowl, add kiwi, maple syrup, and vanilla and stir. Mix in oats, salt, and peanuts. Pour into a greased baking dish and bake for 25-30 minutes, until crisp. Let completely cool and slice into bars to serve

255) SPECIAL TROPICAL CHEESECAKE

Preparation Time: 20 minutes + cooling time

Servings: 4

Ingredients:
- 2/3 cup toasted rolled oats
- ¼ cup plant butter, melted
- 3 tbsp pure date sugar
- 6 oz cashew cream cheese
- ¼ cup coconut milk
- 1 lemon, zested and juiced
- ¼ cup just-boiled water
- 3 tsp agar agar powder
- 1 ripe mango, chopped

Directions:
- Process the oats, butter, and date sugar in a blender until smooth.
- Pour the mixture into a greased 9-inch springform pan and press the mixture onto the bottom of the pan. Refrigerate for 30 minutes until firm while you make the filling.
- In a large bowl, using an electric mixer, whisk the cashew cream cheese until smooth. Beat in the coconut milk, lemon zest, and lemon juice. Mix the boiled water and agar agar powder until dissolved and whisk this mixture into the creamy mix. Fold in the mango.
- Remove the cake pan from the fridge and pour in the mango mixture. Shake the pan to ensure a smooth layering on top. Refrigerate further for at least 3 hours. Remove the cheesecake from the fridge, release the cake pan, slice, and serve

256) ENGLISH RAISIN OATMEAL BISCUITS

Preparation Time: 20 minutes

Servings: 8

Ingredients:
- ½ cup plant butter
- 1 cup date sugar
- ¼ cup pineapple juice
- 1 cup whole-grain flour
- 1 tsp baking powder
- ½ tsp salt
- 1 tsp pure vanilla extract
- 1 cup old-fashioned oats
- ½ cup vegan chocolate chips
- ½ cup raisins

Directions:
- Preheat oven to 370 F. Beat the butter and sugar in a bowl until creamy and fluffy. Pour in the juice and blend. Mix in flour, baking powder, salt, and vanilla. Stir in oats, chocolate chips, and raisins. Spread the dough on a baking sheet and bake for 15 minutes. Let completely cool on a rack

257) EXOTIC COCONUT AND CHOCOLATE BROWNIES

Preparation Time: 40 minutes | | **Servings:** 4

Ingredients:
- 1 cup whole-grain flour
- ½ cup unsweetened cocoa powder
- 1 tsp baking powder
- ½ tsp salt
- 1 cup pure date sugar
- ½ cup canola oil
- ¾ cup almond milk
- 1 tsp pure vanilla extract
- 1 tsp coconut extract
- ½ cup vegan chocolate chips
- ½ cup sweetened shredded coconut

- Preheat oven to 360 F. In a bowl, combine the flour, cocoa, baking powder, and salt.
- In another bowl, whisk the date sugar and oil until creamy. Add in almond milk, vanilla, and coconut extracts. Mix until smooth. Pour into the flour mixture and stir to combine. Fold in the coconut and chocolate chips. Pour the batter into a greased baking pan and bake for 35-40 minutes. Let cool before serving

258) RICH EVERYDAY ENERGY BARS

Preparation Time: 35 minutes | | **Servings:** 16

Ingredients:
- 1 cup vegan butter
- 1 cup brown sugar
- 2 tbsp agave syrup
- 2 cups old-fashioned oats
- 1/2 cup almonds, slivered
- 1/2 cup walnuts, chopped
- 1/2 cup dried currants
- 1/2 cup pepitas

- Begin by preheating your oven to 320 degrees F. Line a baking pan with parchment paper or Silpat mat.
- Thoroughly combine all the ingredients until everything is well incorporated.
- Spread the mixture onto the prepared baking pan using a wide spatula.
- Bake for about 33 minutes or until golden brown. Cut into bars using a sharp knife and enjoy

259) HEALTHY RAW COCONUT ICE CREAM

Preparation Time: 10 minutes + chilling time | | **Servings:** 2

Ingredients:
- 4 over-ripe bananas, frozen
- 4 tbsp coconut milk
- 6 fresh dates, pitted
- 1/4 tsp pure coconut extract
- 1/2 tsp pure vanilla extract
- 1/2 cup coconut flakes

- Place all the ingredients in the bowl of your food processor or high-speed blender.
- Blitz the ingredients until creamy or until your desired consistency is achieved.
- Serve immediately or store in your freezer.
- Enjoy

260) DELICIOUS CHOCOLATE HAZELNUT FUDGE

Preparation Time: 1 hour 10 minutes | | **Servings:** 20

Ingredients:
- 1 cup cashew butter
- 1 cup fresh dates, pitted
- 1/4 cup cocoa powder
- 1/4 tsp ground cloves
- 1 tsp matcha powder
- 1 tsp vanilla extract
- 1/2 cup hazelnuts, coarsely chopped

- Process all ingredients in your blender until uniform and smooth.
- Scrape the batter into a parchment-lined baking sheet. Place it in your freezer for at least 1 hour to set.
- Cut into squares and serve. Enjoy

261) ENGLISH OATMEAL SQUARES WITH CRANBERRIES

Preparation Time: 25 minutes | | **Servings:** 20

Ingredients:
- 1 ½ cups rolled oats
- 1/2 cup brown sugar
- 1 tsp baking soda
- A pinch of coarse salt
- A pinch of grated nutmeg
- 1/2 tsp cinnamon
- 2/3 cup peanut butter
- 1 medium banana, mashed
- 1/3 cup oat milk
- 1 tsp vanilla extract
- 1/2 cup dried cranberries

- Begin by preheating your oven to 350 degrees F.
- In a mixing bowl, thoroughly combine the dry ingredients. In another bowl, combine the wet ingredients.
- Then, stir the wet mixture into the dry ingredients; mix to combine well.
- Spread the batter mixture in a parchment-lined baking pan. Bake in the preheated oven for about 20 minutes.
- Let it cool on a wire rack. Cut into squares and enjoy

Bibliography

FROM THE SAME AUTHOR

PLANT-BASED DIET FOR MEN Cookbook - The Best 120+ High-Protein Green Meals! Make your body STRONG and FIT with the Healthiest Recipes for Him!

PLANT-BASED DIET FOR WOMEN Cookbook - More than 120 High-Protein Recipes to stay TONE and have more ENERGY! Start your Green Lifestyle with one of the Healthiest Diet for Her Overall!

PLANT-BASED DIET Cookbook - The Best 120+ Green Recipes for a healthier Lifestyle! Stay FIT and have more ENERGY with many High-Protein Vegan and Vegetarian Meals!

PLANT-BASED COOKBOOK FOR STUDENTS - FOCUS ON STUDYING - The Best 120+ Recipes to Stay more CONCENTRATED and have more ENERGY! Maintain Perfect your Focus on Studying with many High-Protein Vegan and Vegetarian Meals!

PLANT-BASED DIET FOR COUPLE Cookbook - More than 220 High-Protein Vegetarian Recipes to Surprise your Partner in the Kitchen! Start your Healthier Lifestyle with the Best Green Meals to Make Together!

HIGH PROTEIN PLANT-BASED COOKBOOK FOR ATHLETES - Many High-Protein Vegan and Vegetarian Recipes to Boost your Body to the TOP! The Best 220+ Green and Healthy Recipes to Perform your Muscles and Sculpt your Abs stay LIGHT!

PLANT-BASED DIET FOR HEALTHY MUM & KIDS Cookbook - The Best 220+ Green Recipes to make with your Kids! Start a HAPPY and HEALTHY Lifestyle with the Quickest Vegetarian and Vegan Recipes for your Family!

QUICK AND EASY PLANT-BASED DIET Cookbook - The Simplest and Quickest High-Protein Green Recipes to Start Your Healthy Lifestyle! Stay LIGHT cooking More Than 220+ Very Easy Meals Without Stress!

PLANT-BASED DIET FOR FITNESS WOMAN Cookbook - More than 220 Super Healthy Vegan and Vegetarian Recipes to Increase your Energy, Detox Your Body, and Improve your Body Tone to the TOP! Stay FIT and LIGHT with these Best Selected High-Protein Green Meals!

PLANT-BASED FOR YOUNG ATHLETES Cookbook - Many Green and Healthy Recipes to Perform your Body Tone while stay LIGHT! The Best 220+ High-Protein Vegetarian Recipes to stay Fit and Start a New Lifestyle!

Conclusion

Thanks for reading "The High-Protein Plant-Based Cookbook for Athletes"!

Follow the right habits it is essential to have a healthy Lifestyle, and the Plant-Based diet is the best solution!

I hope you liked this Cookbook and I wish you to achieve all your goal!

William Miller

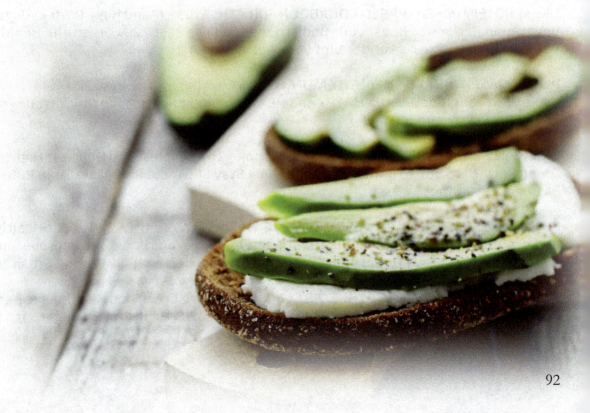

CPSIA information can be obtained
at www.ICGtesting.com
Printed in the USA
BVHW051638140621
609528BV00009B/1302